April–September 2006 Volume 6 Numbers 2 & 3 Pages 117–272

Parenting: Science and Practice

This journal is abstracted or indexed in *PsycINFO/Psychological Abstracts; Cumulative Index to Nursing and Allied Health Literature (CINAHL); EBSCOhost Products; Family & Society Studies Worldwide; Cabell's Directory of Publishing Opportunities in Psychology; Family Index Database.*

First published 2006 by Lawrence Erlbaum Associates, Inc.

2 Park Square, Milton Park, Abingdon, Oxfordshire OX14 4RN
52 Vanderbilt Avenue, New York, NY 10017

Routledge is an imprint of the Taylor & Francis Group, an informa business

First issued in hardback 2019

ISBN 13: 978-0-8058-9380-9 (pbk)
ISBN 13: 978-1-138-40862-3 (hbk)

PARENTING: SCIENCE AND PRACTICE April–September 2006 Volume 6 Numbers 2 & 3 Pages 117–143

The Early Head Start Father Studies: Design, Data Collection, and Summary of Father Presence in the Lives of Infants and Toddlers

Kimberly Boller, Robert Bradley, Natasha Cabrera, Helen H. Raikes, Barbara Pan, Jeffrey Shears, and Lori Roggman

SYNOPSIS

In this introductory article to the Special Issue, we provide an overview of the research and policy context for the Early Head Start Father Studies. We describe the methods used to conduct the father studies, which began in 1997 and were designed to complement the Early Head Start Research and Evaluation Project, a random assignment evaluation of 3,001 families — half who received Early Head Start services and half who did not. The Early Head Start Father Studies included in the Special Issue addressed 5 key research questions about low-income fathers and their children (all under 3 years old) using a variety of data collection approaches, including mother report, father report, father – child videotaped interactions, and Early Head Start program staff report. Here we describe the father studies' methods and response rates, father demographics, and father – child relationship status.

INTRODUCTION

Research Context for Studies of Low-Income Fathers and Their Role in Young Children's Lives

The literature on fatherhood consistently associates father absence with maladjustment, low competence, and poor life choices in children (Federal Interagency Forum on Child and Family Statistics, 1998). Boys growing up without fathers seem especially prone to problems in the areas of sex-role and gender-identity development, school performance, psychosocial adjustment, and self-control (Hetherington & Stanley-Hagan, 1986). Girls are affected by father absence as well, although the effects may be less enduring, dramatic, and pervasive than those for boys. Girls growing up without a father are at risk for early sexual activity and adolescent pregnancy (Ellis et al., 2003; McLanahan & Sandefur, 1994; Newcomer & Udry, 1987). By contrast, positive father involvement (i.e., warm, stimulating, engaged, and responsible fathering) is often associated with positive outcomes for children (Lamb, 1997; Lewis, 1997; Parke, 2002; Shannon, Tamis-LeMonda, London, & Cabrera, 2002; Tamis-LeMonda, Shannon, Cabrera, & Lamb, 2004). Paternal involvement can influence children's outcomes directly. It can also influence child well-being indirectly via its influence on maternal parenting and the building of social networks (Clarke-Stewart, 1978; Lamb, 1997; Lewis, Feiring, & Weinraub, 1981; Lewis & Weinraub, 1976).

These general patterns acknowledged, not having a father does not inevitably lead to serious negative consequences for children (Lamb, 1999). Likewise, the mere presence of a father does not guarantee good outcomes. The information available on nonresident fathers is especially difficult to interpret. Part of the difficulty derives from the fact that nonresident fathers vary greatly in terms of involvement and commitment to their children. Some studies show no relation between nonresident father involvement and children's outcomes, but other research suggests that beneficial effects on children can occur under certain circumstances (e.g., when there exists a positive father – mother relationship). Moreover, sometimes when fathers are present in the home, family conflict is also evident. Conflict and hostility between parents can have deleterious effects on children's socioemotional well-being and behavior (Amato, 1993; Cherlin et al., 1991; Cummings & O'Reilly, 1997; Fincham, 1998). When fathers are unsupportive and marital conflict is high, children may suffer (Cummings & O'Reilly, 1997; Goeke-Morey & Cummings, 2005).

Despite three decades of rather intensive research on fathers, the picture of father involvement is both incomplete and somewhat ambiguous (Cabrera et al., 2000; Coley, 2001; Hernandez & Brandon, 2002). Much about father involvement in low-income families remains unclear. Especially unclear is how that involvement may reflect the father's broader set of involvements in social institutions. This Special Issue attempts to add definition and texture to understanding the nature and consequences of fathering in low-income families.

In designing the father studies component of the Early Head Start National Evaluation Study, we began with several concerns, namely that research on fatherhood has (1) mostly relied on measures of father involvement that are based on a maternal template, (2) not sufficiently considered ethnic and cultural variations in both the type and nature of fatherhood, and (3) lacked a comprehensive theoretical framework to guide researchers in their search for associations between aspects of father involvement and measures of child well-being (Cabrera et al., 2002; Roggman, Fitzgerald, Bradley, & Raikes, 2002). An additional limitation of current knowledge is that the bulk of the research on residential fathers is based on European American middle-class samples; thus, findings cannot readily be generalized to other groups of fathers. In contrast, research on nonresident fathers has used one-dimensional definitions of father involvement such as payment of child support. The limited research on low-income fathers has been conducted from a deficit perspective that reinforces negative stereotypes and neglects within-group variation (McAdoo, 1993; McLoyd, 1998; McLoyd, Cauce, Takeuchi, & Wilson, 2000).

As part of the Early Head Start National Evaluation, we engaged in a series of data collections aimed at better understanding how fathers function in low-income families and how participation in Early Head Start programs may affect fathers' involvement in family life. To this end, data were collected from mothers about fathers and from fathers themselves. Our father involvement interview questionnaire tapped key dimensions of parenting and parent – child relationships. Some of the measures were identical (or nearly identical) to those we used with mothers as part of the larger Early Head Start study. Other measures were unique to fathers. In this process, we attempted to go beyond the "mother template" of good parenting by assessing areas seen as especially salient to fathering and by approaching issues in ways more attuned to a male perspective (Doherty et al., 1998). Central to our conceptualization was a multidimensional definition of father involvement that included information on (1) activities that fathers engage in with their children, (2) how fathers express responsibility for their children, and (3) the types of social, human, and financial capital that fathers afford their children. We also asked fathers several open-ended questions designed to shed light on how men perceive the father role, their experiences with their own fathers, and the support they need to be a father. In addition, we videotaped interactions between fathers and their children.

The Early Head Start Father Studies were designed to be sensitive to the changing nature of the father – child relationship from infancy through early childhood. Additionally, they were targeted to determine the impact of fathering on children's social, emotional, physical, and cognitive development. The study also included a survey of how Early Head Start programs involve fathers in their activities. This aspect of the father studies represented the first large-scale effort aimed at understanding these processes. Information on program involvement was considered especially important given the major shifts in social and governmental policies pertaining to poor families that have emerged in the last decade.

Program and Policy Context

The 1994 congressional Head Start Act included a provision requiring that an evaluation be conducted on the newly authorized Early Head Start program, emphasizing the need for research on its efficacy (for additional background on Early Head Start, see Department of Health and Human Services, 1994). As a result, an evaluation study was commenced during the first year of the program's implementation. The National Early Head Start Research and Evaluation Project has fulfilled multiple purposes, including a national study of implementation (see Administration for Children and Families [ACF], 2002c; Administration on Children, Youth, and Families [ACYF], 1999, 2000) and impacts (ACF, 2002a; ACYF, 2001). Additional funds were also provided to conduct local research on mediators and moderators of program implementation and impacts (for example, local studies of child language development, child nutrition, and attachment) as well as research to inform continuous program improvement (see ACF, 2004a, 2004b). In addition, the National Evaluation features cross-site studies by workgroups, one of which is the Father Studies Workgroup. The workgroups have produced numerous scholarly articles focusing on parenting and the early development of low-income children (e.g., Ispa et al., 2004).

In sum, Early Head Start Father Studies originated in the context of the national program evaluation and its accompanying research agenda. Funding for this effort was provided by the ACYF of the U.S. Department of Health and Human Services, the National Institute for Child Health and Human Development, the Office of the Assistant Secretary for Planning and Evaluation, and the Ford Foundation. Members of the Early Head Start national evaluation study team were joined by representatives from each of these funding agencies in helping to direct the father studies embedded in the larger evaluation study.

Two important national policy changes, namely Welfare Reform and the Federal Fatherhood Initiative, also helped shape the Early Head Start Father Studies. The phenomenon of a "fatherless America" became a popular topic of debate during the 1990s. Children growing up without a father in the household were assumed to grow up "fatherless," without their biological fathers taking financial or any other responsibility for them. Rising crime, family instability, child poverty, juvenile delinquency, and the weakening of men's roles in the family were seen as direct consequences of men's absence from their families. Children living in female-headed households were assumed to have fathers who were uninvolved. This assumption has been questioned, however, on the grounds that national surveys tend to undercount men in nontraditional households (Cherlin & Griffin, 1998). Undercount rates are reported to be higher for nonresident and unmarried fathers, especially minorities, fathers who have unstable housing, never-married fathers, and men who are incarcerated or in the military (Cherlin & Griffin, 1998; Martin & Siegel, 1998; Western & McLanahan, 2000). This undercount of fathers contributed to the public image that low-income, nonresidential fathers were "deadbeats."

The undercount problem had a palpable effect on public policy because of the large number of single mothers on welfare and the substantial amount of uncollected child support (Duncan & Brooks-Gunn, 1997; Edin & Lein, 1997; Garfinkel, McLanahan, & Hanson, 1998). Under the new welfare reform legislation — the 1996 Personal Responsibility and Work Opportunity Reconciliation Act — a block grant called Temporary Assistance for Needy Families (TANF) provides funds to states to run their own programs. Mothers who receive TANF are mandated to enter the workforce even when their children are very young, and nonresident fathers are required to establish paternity for children born out of wedlock and to pay child support without explicit rights to visitation (Cabrera & Peters, 1999). Under the current welfare reform law, mothers can lose their benefits if they do not provide information about the father of their child (Cabrera & Evans, 2000). Recent findings suggest that child support enforcement, after paternity has been established, is the most important governmental tool to increase nonresident father involvement (Sorensen & Pomper, 2003).

At the same time, the "missing men" problem had an impact at the federal level and became the highlight of a major federal initiative, the 1996 to 1997 Fatherhood Research Initiative, that led to a reorganization of the way that many federally funded initiatives collect data on fathers and families (Cabrera et al., 2002). This initiative specifically included a federal mandate to involve men and fathers in research, programs, and services. One recommendation of the Fatherhood Research Initiative was to use the Early Head Start Research and Evaluation Project as a laboratory for conducting basic theoretical research on the meaning and nature of fathering for low-income men and their children (Cabrera et al., 2002). The Early Head Start Father Studies became part of a trio of studies, along with the Fragile Families and Child Well-Being Study (Carlson, McLanahan, & Brooks-Gunn, 2005; Reichman, Teitler, Garfinkel, &

McLanahan, 2001) and the Early Childhood Longitudinal Birth Cohort study, designed to produce new data on how men father, the investments they make on behalf of their children, the determinants of father involvement, the influence of this involvement on their children's development, and the barriers and challenges fathers face. Although these studies vary in terms of design, purpose, and population, the measures used to assess father involvement share commonalities of constructs and survey questions (see Cabrera et al., 2004, for a comparison of the fatherhood measures included in these three large-scale surveys). (For relevant findings from the Fragile Families and Child Well-Being Study, see Carlson & McLanahan, 2002; Hijjawi, Wilson, & Turkheimer, 2003; Kalil, 2003; Wilson & Brooks-Gunn, 2001.)

The remaining sections of this introductory article provide an overview of the project methods and research questions pertaining to fathers and their families in the Early Head Start Research and Evaluation. After reviewing the key aspects of each data collection approach and the father study research questions, we highlight the specific articles in this Special Issue that address them.

STUDY METHODS

Main Study

In 1995, ACF selected 17 programs to participate in the national evaluation of Early Head Start (referred to here as the Main Study). The 17 sites in the Main Study are located in urban and rural settings across the country. A total of 3,001 families applying to these Early Head Start programs between July 1996 and September 1998 were randomly assigned either to the program (1,513) or to a control (1,488) group. Families assigned to the control group could access all services in the community except Early Head Start. The samples in most sites included between 150 and 200 families, divided fairly evenly between the program and control groups. Early Head Start research families were diverse: 63% were either Latin American, African American, or belonged to other non-European American groups. Forty-eight percent of parents had not earned a high school diploma, 39% were teenage parents, and 55% were neither employed nor in school. See Table 1 for a summary of sample characteristics at the time of program enrollment (baseline). Families were offered modest remuneration and a small gift to complete each set of interviews and assessments. Ninety-five percent of the 3,001 primary caregivers who

TABLE 1
Main Study Primary Caregiver, Household, and Child Characteristics at Baseline

	Sample Size	Percentage of Families
Parent and family characteristics		
Mother's age at birth of focus child		
Less than 20	1,142	39
20 or older	1,771	61
Missing	88	
Mother's age at birth of first child		
Less than 19	1,247	42
19 or older	1,720	58
Missing	34	
Mother's education		
Less than grade 12	1,375	48
Grade 12 or attained a GED	822	29
Greater than grade 12	682	24
Missing	122	
Race and ethnicity		
European American	1,091	37
African American Non-Latin American	1,014	35
Latin American	693	24
Other	135	5
Missing	68	
Primary occupation		
Employed	677	24
In school or training	630	22
Neither	1,590	55
Missing	104	
Primary language		
English	2,265	79
Other	615	21
Missing	121	
Living arrangements		
With spouse	752	25
With other adults	1,157	39
Alone with child(ren)	1,080	36
Missing	12	
Presence of adult male in the household		
Male present	1,153	39
Male not present	1,836	61
Missing	12	
Focus child characteristics		
Age		
Unborn	761	25
Less than 5 months	1,063	35
5 months or older	1,177	39
Missing	0	

(continued)

Table 1 *(Continued)*

	Sample Size	Percentage of Families
Gender		
Boy	1,510	51
Girl	1,448	49
Missing	43	
First born		
Yes	1,858	63
No	1,112	37
Missing	31	
Sample size	3,001	

Note. Adapted from Administration for Children and Families (2002a). Data are from Head Start Family Information System application and enrollment forms completed prior to random assignment. GED = government equivalency diploma.

were enrolled in the study and were subsequently targeted for parent interviews were mothers. In 1997, data collection was expanded in the research sites to include fathers. (See ACF, 2002a, and Love et al., 2005, for reports pertaining to the impact of Early Head Start on child outcomes and family functioning.)

Data on family demographics and service needs were collected prior to random assignment. Analyses of these baseline data demonstrated that random assignment was successful in yielding two very similar groups, and that any differences observed after baseline could be ascribed to the Early Head Start intervention. Families were subsequently interviewed about service use at 6, 15, and 26 months after random assignment and at the conclusion of the Main Study. Interviews with primary caregivers (usually mothers), videotaped parent – child interaction, and assessments of children's development were conducted when the children were approximately 14, 24, and 36 months old. Data collectors in each site were trained and certified using a common set of procedures (see ACF, 2002b, for details).

Mothers were asked during the interviews about the child's biological father and his involvement with the child. If the biological father did not live with the mother and child, mothers were asked about any man in the child's life who was "like a father" to the child. At the end of the interview, researchers informed mothers about the father study and asked mothers for their help in setting up an interview with the identified father or father figure who was most involved in the child's life.

A wide variety of outcome measures was collected as part of the parent interview and the direct child assessments. Selected categories of outcome measures from the Main Study and their data sources are summarized in Table 2. Table 3 displays overall response rates for key data sources. Interview respondents were participants who provided data that could be used to construct key outcome variables. Nonrespondents include those who could not be located as well as those who could be located but for whom complete or usable data were not obtained.

Based on maternal reports, close to 90% of children in the study had some contact with either their biological father or a father figure (see Table 4 and ACF, 2002a) at age 36 months. Mothers reported that almost 72% of children lived with or had contact at least a few times per month with their biological fathers. These rates of father presence were consistent with earlier mother reports when the children were 14 and 24 months old. (See Cabrera et al., 2004, for an in-depth presentation of father involvement at 24 months.)

Forty percent of mothers at child age 36 months reported that they were married, a substantial increase over the 26% who reported being married at study entry (not shown in Table 4). Of these, just over a third were married to the child's biological father. In total, about half of the mothers reported being either married to, living with, or in a romantic relationship with the child's biological father at child age 3 (not shown in Table 4).

Overall, families in the Early Head Start group and the control group were comparable in their mother-reported rates of biological father or male presence — the program did not affect these rates through 36 months (ACF, 2002a). Fathers themselves reported being involved with their children in a variety of ways; but, overall, Early Head Start had no impact on the types and amounts of involvement fathers had with their children — the frequencies of caregiving, social, cognitive, and physical play activities were comparable across the Early Head Start and the control groups. Early Head Start had impacts on a few important father and father - child behaviors. Fathers whose families were in the Early Head Start group reported less spanking, and they were coded as less intrusive during play with their children than control-group fathers. In addition, children of fathers in the Early Head Start group were more likely to engage the father and to demonstrate sustained attention with objects than were children of fathers in the control group. (Of the studies reported in this Special Issue, the following draw data from the Main Study: Fitzgerald, McKelvey, Schiffman, & Montañez; Ryan, Martin, & Brooks-Gunn; Vogel, Bradley, Raikes, Bollet, & Shears.)

TABLE 2
Main Study Selected Categories of Early Head Start Outcome Variables and Their Data Sources

Outcome Measure	Data Source
Parenting behavior, knowledge, and the home environment	
Knowledge of child development, discipline strategies, and safety precautions	14-, 24-, and 36-month parent interviews
Parent supportiveness, detachment, intrusiveness, and negative regard	Coding from videotaped parent – child semistructured play task (14, 24, and 36 months)
Parent quality of assistance, detachment, and intrusiveness	Coding from videotaped puzzle challenge task (36 months)
Parent warmth, harshness, and stimulation of language and learning	14-, 24-, and 36-month parent interviews
Quality of cognitive and emotional support provided in the home environment	14-, 24-, and 36-month parent interviews and interviewer observations
Child development	
Child social and emotional well-being	
Child engagement, negativity toward parent, and sustained attention with objects	Coding from videotaped parent – child semistructured play task (14, 24, and 36 months)
Child engagement, persistence, and frustration	Coding from videotaped puzzle challenge task (36 months)
Emotional regulation, orientation, and engagement	Interviewer observations (14, 24, and 36 months)
Aggressive behavior	14-, 24-, and 36-month parent interviews
Child cognitive and language development	
Bayley Mental Development Index (MDI)	Direct child assessment (14, 24, and 36 months)
Vocabulary production and sentence complexity	14- and 24-month parent interviews
Receptive vocabulary	Direct child assessment (36 months)
Child health status	14-, 24-, and 36-month parent interviews
Family outcomes	
Mother's health and mental health	
Depression	14-, 24-, and 36-month parent interviews
Parenting stress	14-, 24-, and 36-month parent interviews
Family functioning	
Family conflict	14-, 24-, and 36-month parent interviews
Self-sufficiency	
Education and training	6-, 15-, and 26-month parent services interviews
Welfare receipt	6-, 15-, and 26-month parent services interviews
Employment and income	6-, 15-, and 26-month parent services interviews
Father characteristics, presence and behavior	
Father education and employment	14-, 24-, and 36-month parent interviews
Father presence	14-, 24-, and 36-month parent interviews
Father activities with child	14-, 24-, and 36-month parent interviews

Note. Adapted from Administration for Children and Families (2002a).

TABLE 3
Main Study Response Rates
to Key Parent Interview
and Child Assessment Data Sources

Data Source	Percentage
Parent service interviews	
6-month	81.6
15-month	75.2
26-month	69.5
15- and 26-month	61.5
All three	56.5
Parent interviews	
14-month	78.1
24-month	72.2
36-month	70.3
24- and 36-month	61.4
All three	56.7
Bayley assessments	
14-month	62.7
24-month	59.4
36-month	55.0
24- and 36-month	43.6
All three	34.8
Sample size	3,001

Note. Adapted from Administration for Children and Families (2002a).

Father Involvement With Toddlers Substudy (FITS)

Twelve of the seventeen research sites elected to participate in a series of studies of the fathers of focus children in the Main Study. These sites were located in Arkansas, Colorado (2 sites), Iowa, Michigan, New York, Pennsylvania, Tennessee, Utah, Vermont, and Washington (2 sites). In these sites, at the end of the 24- and 36-month interview with the mother, the interviewer described the father study, reviewed the father interview section, and identified the man most involved with the child. Approximately 76% of the completed mother interviews at child age 24 months at the FITS sites yielded a viable father interview identification. Of those who were identified, researchers were able to interview 727, or 62%. Approximately half the interviews were completed with fathers of children in the program group, the other half with fathers of children in the control group. At child age 36 months, 73% of interviewed mothers identified a father or father fig-

TABLE 4
Main Study Father Relationship, Residence, and Involvement as Reported by Mothers When Children were 14, 24, and 36 Months Old by Race and Ethnicity

	14 Months			24 Months			36 Months		
	N	Percentage	*SD*	*N*	Percentage	*SD*	*N*	Percentage	*SD*
Resident biological father									
Overall	616	30	0.46	631	31	0.46	717	35	0.48
European American	298	38	0.49	307	39	0.49	335	43	0.50
African American	74	11	0.31	73	11	0.31	86	13	0.34
Latin American	191	41	0.49	204	44	0.50	244	53	0.50
Other	37	44	0.50	34	40	0.49	37	44	0.50
Married resident biological father									
Overall	268	13	0.34	217	11	0.31	208	10	0.30
European American	118	15	0.36	88	11	0.32	81	10	0.30
African American	73	11	0.31	57	09	0.28	57	09	0.28
Latin American	61	13	0.34	55	12	0.32	55	12	0.32
Other	12	14	0.35	10	12	0.33	10	12	0.33
Biological father present (Resident or contact a few times per month or more)									
Overall	1,326	77	0.42	1,278	75	0.43	1,406	72	0.45
European American	538	79	0.41	518	76	0.43	542	72	0.45
African American	388	70	0.46	354	67	0.47	422	66	0.47
Latin American	311	84	0.37	320	84	0.37	352	81	0.39
Other	61	82	0.38	59	87	0.34	63	78	0.42
Man (Biological father or father figure) present									
Overall	1,572	90	0.30	1,579	90	0.30	1,793	89	0.31
European American	629	91	0.28	636	92	0.28	700	91	0.29
African American	486	86	0.34	481	87	0.34	562	85	0.36
Latin American	354	93	0.26	362	91	0.29	418	93	0.26
Other	71	93	0.25	68	94	0.23	78	95	0.22

Note. Parent interviews were conducted when children were approximately 14, 24, and 36 months old. Categories presented here are not mutually exclusive, thus, column percentages do not total 100.

ure, of whom 698, or 64%, completed the father interview. See Table 5 for FITS sample sizes and response rates by site. Interviewed fathers were ethnically and racially diverse.

At both the 24- and 36-month interviews, almost two thirds of the interviewed men were resident biological fathers (64.2% and 61.5%, respectively; see Table 6). Nonresident biological fathers (16.4% at 24 months and 15.0% at 36 months) and resident father figures (15.6% at 24 months and 17.9% at 36 months) made up the remaining one third of the sample. Nonresident father figures constituted a very small proportion of the men interviewed; for this reason, most of the studies in this Special Issue did not

TABLE 5
FITS Father Interview Sample Sizes and Response Rates for Program and Control Groups by Site[a]

	Father Interviews			
Site	24-Month Sample Size	Response Rate[b] (Percentage)	36-Month Sample Size	Response Rate[b] (Percentage)
1	51	45	44	37
3	54	45	30	25
4	63	57	52	46
6	36	24	55	40
8	83	55	96	66
10	47	51	44	52
11	30	25	37	27
13	102	69	101	69
14	48	44	44	44
15	71	54	53	43
16	74	50	82	59
17	68	46	60	44
Total	727	62	698	64

Note. Adapted with permission from Administration for Children and Families (2002b). FITS = Father Involvement with Toddlers Substudy.

[a]Two additional sites, California and Missouri, began the father study but ended their participation after completing 34 (20 in California and 14 in Missouri) 24-month interviews and 9 (2 in California and 7 in Missouri) 36-month interviews. In addition, because few nonresident father figures were identified and completed the father interviews, they were dropped from the response rate analyses for FITS and from most of the subsequent analyses. One study described in this Special Issue (Summers, Boller, Schiffman, & Raikes) used data from these two sites and included data from nonresident father figures. The other studies did not.

[b]The response rate was calculated by using the number of fathers identified by mothers during the 24- or 36-month parent interviews as the denominator.

TABLE 6
FITS Father Relationship and Residence Status as Reported by Fathers at 24 and 36 Months by Race and Ethnicity

	24 Months			36 Months		
	N	Percentage	*SD*	*N*	Percentage	*SD*
Resident biological father						
Overall	494	64	0.48	455	62	0.49
European American	97	80	0.41	112	73	0.45
African American	47	46	0.50	66	43	0.50
Latin American	181	73	0.44	208	65	0.48
Other	15	79	0.42	19	63	0.49
Nonresident biological father						
Overall	126	16	0.37	111	15	0.36
European American	13	11	0.31	12	08	0.27
African American	29	28	0.45	44	29	0.45
Latin American	28	11	0.32	42	13	0.34
Other	0	00	0.00	3	10	0.31
Resident father figure						
Overall	120	16	0.36	132	18	0.38
European American	10	08	0.28	22	14	0.35
African American	20	20	0.40	32	21	0.41
Latin American	30	12	0.33	57	18	0.38
Other	3	16	0.37	6	20	0.41
Nonresident father figure						
Overall	29	04	0.19	41	06	0.23
European American	2	02	0.13	8	05	0.22
African American	6	06	0.24	12	08	0.27
Latin American	8	03	0.18	13	04	0.20
Other	1	05	0.23	2	07	0.25

Note. Father interviews were conducted when children were approximately 24 and 36 months old. Columns do not add to overall totals because of missing data for father race and ethnicity. FITS = Father Involvement with Toddlers Substudy.

include nonresident fathers in their analyses because of concerns about small cell sizes ($n = 29$ at 24 months and $n = 41$ at 36 months).

The fathers and father figures in the sample were about 27 years old on average when the focus child was born. Most of the men were employed either part or full time (89% at 24 months and 92% at 36 months). On average, the men had just less than 12 years of education.

In addition to demographic information, father interviews asked about parenting stress, depression, and stressful life events fathers experienced; fathers' beliefs about fathering, their fathering experiences, and their experiences with their own parents; and their relationships with their child, the child's mother, and other relatives. Table 7 summarizes the main areas included in the father interviews.

Fathers and father figures who completed the interview differed systematically from those who did not. Compared with the sample of identified nonrespondents, fathers who completed the FITS interviews were more likely to be resident biological fathers, married to the child's mother, and generally more advantaged (ACF, 2002b; Cabrera et al., 2004). Thus, findings about the interviewed group may not generalize to the larger sample of fathers and father figures in the Main Study or to the population of families eligible for Early Head Start. We return to the implications of these response analyses in the final article (Bradley, Shears, Roggman, & Tamis-LeMonda, this issue). (Of the reports in this Special Issue, the fol-

TABLE 7
FITS Selected Categories of Early Head Start 24- and 36-Month Outcome Variables

Outcome Measure
Father behavior and knowledge
Father caregiving, social, cognitive, and physical play activities
Knowledge of child development
Father discipline strategies
Index of severity of discipline strategies
Spanked child in previous week
Father roles and attitudes
Fathering role perceptions
Father investment in child
Father role in child-related decisions
Father relationships
Experiences with his parents
Quality of relationship with child's mother
Quality of relationship with family (his and mother's)
Father well being
Father's mental health
Depression
Parenting stress
Family Functioning
Family conflict
Father self-sufficiency
Education and training
Employment and income

Note. Adapted from Administration for Children and Families (2002b). FITS = Father Involvement with Toddlers Substudy.

lowing drew data from FITS: Fitzgerald et al.; Ryan et al.; Summers, Boller, Schiffman, & Raikes.)

Fathers of Toddlers Qualitative Interview Substudy (FTQIS)

This study was based on analysis of audiotaped, open-ended questions embedded in the FITS father interviews at child ages 24 and 36 months. Accounting for tapes that were inaudible or defective, the total sample represented in the FTQIS was 575 fathers and father figures at 24 months. An average of 41 fathers participated (ranging from 9 to 67) from each of the 14 sites.[1] Sixty-six percent were resident biological fathers, 16% were nonresident biological fathers, 15% were resident father figures (such as the child's grandfather or the mother's husband or partner), and 4% were nonresident father figures (with rounding, the total is greater than 100%). The FTQIS sample was demographically comparable at 36 months.

The qualitative interview protocol for the 24- and 36-month interview included six primary or "grand tour" items (Miles & Huberman, 1994): (1) What does being a "good father" mean to you? (2) How has becoming a father impacted your life? (3) Talk about your experiences with your own father. (4) What kinds of help or support do you get to do your job as a father? (5) What gets in the way of being a father? (6) What are you proudest of about your child? The Father Studies Workgroup developed a series of suggested probes related to each grand tour question to serve as guidelines for the interviewers and intended to elicit more elaborative responses to these questions. (The study reported by Summers et al., this issue, used data from FTQIS and addresses qualitative question 1. See Summers, Boller, & Raikes, 2004, for related reports.)

Father and Child Interaction During Toddlerhood Substudy (FACITS)

This substudy involved data collected at 9 of the 12 FITS sites. Father–child interaction was videotaped when the children were 24 (n = 339) and 36 (n = 340) months of age. Table 8 summarizes the father relation-

[1]This study included the two additional father study sites described earlier (CA and MO) and included nonresident father figures.

TABLE 8
FACITS Father Relationship and Residence Status as Reported by Fathers at 24 and 36 Months by Race and Ethnicity

	24 Months			36 Months		
	N	Percentage	*SD*	*N*	Percentage	*SD*
Resident biological father						
Overall	230	68	0.47	219	64	0.48
European American	110	81	0.39	126	74	0.44
African American	31	53	0.50	42	48	0.50
Latin American	16	64	0.49	18	55	0.51
Other	10	77	0.44	13	72	0.46
Nonresident biological father						
Overall	52	15	0.36	49	14	0.35
European American	9	07	0.25	15	09	0.28
African American	18	31	0.46	24	28	0.45
Latin American	5	20	0.41	5	15	0.36
Other	0	00	0.00	1	06	0.24
Resident father figure						
Overall	50	15	0.36	62	18	0.39
European American	13	10	0.30	26	15	0.36
African American	8	14	0.35	17	20	0.40
Latin American	4	16	0.37	9	27	0.45
Other	2	15	0.38	3	17	0.38
Nonresident father figure						
Overall	7	0.02	0.14	10	0.03	0.17
European American	3	0.02	0.15	3	0.02	0.13
African American	2	0.03	0.18	4	0.05	0.21
Latin American	0	0.00	0.00	1	0.03	0.17
Other	1	0.08	0.28	1	0.06	0.24

Note. Father interviews and assessments of father – child interactions conducted when children were 24 and 36 months old. Columns do not add to overall totals because of missing data for father race/ethnicity. FACITS = Father And Child Interaction during Toddlerhood Substudy.

ship and residence status of fathers in this sample overall and by race and ethnicity.

At 24 months, the FACITS assessment activities comprised (1) a Nursing Child Assessment Satellite Training Programs teaching task, (2) a task where fathers chose what they wanted to do ("Your choice"), (3) a semistructured play task with book and toys brought by the interviewer, and (4) a clean-up task. The teaching and semistructured play activities were identical to the mother – child interaction protocol, except that the specific age-appropriate materials were changed so that children would not be bored. To help identify unique dimensions of fathers' interactions with toddlers, the Father Studies Workgroup developed the "Your Choice" task that included asking the fathers to do something for 5 min with their child that they would typically enjoy doing with the child. At 36 months, a problem-solving task with puzzles replaced the teaching task, and the clean-up task was dropped. The types of outcomes coded from the video data are summarized in Table 9. (Ryan et al., this Issue, report findings emerging from analyses of the FACITS data.)

Research Questions Guiding the Early Head Start Father Studies

The research agenda for the Early Head Start Father Studies encompasses a wide range of questions. Articles in this Special Issue are representative of the larger set of studies undertaken as part of the Early Head Start Father Studies research program. Table 10 provides a crosswalk between the articles in this Special Issue and their data sources. Within this Special Issue we attempt to address the following scientific questions.

What is the role of fathers in the lives of low-income children? Given that fewer than half of Early Head Start mothers live with the child's father (ACYF, 2001), the study presented an opportunity to learn more about

TABLE 9
FACITS Selected Categories of Early Head Start Outcome Variables and Their Data Sources

Outcome Measure	Data Source
Father behavior with the child	
Father supportiveness and intrusiveness	Coding from Videotaped Father – Child Semistructured Play Task (24 and 36 months)
Father quality of assistance and intrusiveness	Coding from Videotaped Father – Child Puzzle Challenge Task (36 months)
Child behavior with the father	
Child engagement of the father, negativity toward the father, and sustained attention with objects	Coding from Videotaped Father – Child Semistructured Play Task (24 and 36 months)
Child engagement of father, persistence, and frustration	Coding from Videotaped Father – Child Puzzle Challenge Task (36 months)

Note. Adapted from Administration for Children and Families (2002b). FACITS = Father and Child Interaction during Toddlerhood Study.

TABLE 10
Special Issue Articles and Their Data Sources

Article Title	Data Source
The Meaning of "Good Fatherhood": Low-Income Fathers' Social Constructions of Their Roles (Summers, Boller, Schiffman, & Raikes)	Father Involvement with Toddlers Substudy (FITS) and Fathers of Toddlers Qualitative Interview Substudy
Fathering in Infancy: Mutuality and Stability Between 8 and 16 Months (Shannon, Tamis LeMonda, & Cabrera)	Father and Newborn Study
Relations Between Father Connectedness and Child Outcomes (Vogel, Bradley, Raikes, Boller, & Shears)	Main Study
Is One Good Parent Good Enough? Patterns of Mother and Father Parenting and Child Cognitive Outcomes at 24 and 36 Months (Ryan, Martin, & Brooks-Gunn)	Main Study, FITS, and Father and Child Interaction During Toddlerhood Substudy
Two Studies of Father Involvement in Early Head Start Programs: A National Survey and a Demonstration Program Evaluation (Raikes & Bellotti)	Participation in Fatherhood Programs and Services Use Study and Fatherhood Demonstration Study
Exposure of Low-Income Families and Their Children to Neighborhood Violence and Paternal Antisocial Behavior (Fitzgerald, McKelvey, Schiffman, & Montanez)	Main Study and FITS

both resident and nonresident fathers. It further offered the opportunity to better understand how low-income fathers of all types viewed their roles, responsibilities, and relationships, and the meaning of fatherhood and fertility as well as the perceptions of the stressors and joys of fatherhood. "The Meaning of 'Good Fatherhood:' Low-Income Fathers' Social Constructions of Their Roles," in this Special Issue by Summers et al., analyzes the qualitative responses of fathers about their roles as fathers. When asked what being a "good father" meant to them, men identified four major roles: (1) being a stable figure in the child's life, (2) teaching, (3) interacting physically with the child, and (4) providing emotional support. These fathers also made clear how lack of financial resources and being physically apart from the child impeded their ability to effectively enact these roles.

How do involved, low-income fathers interact with their young children? The Early Head Start Father Studies afforded a rare opportunity to learn more about low-income fathers' engagement with infants using father – child videotaped data. In "Fathering in Infancy: Mutuality and Stability Between 8 and 16 Months," in this Special Issue, Shannon, Tamis-LeMonda, and Cabrera examine the quality of father – child interactions. The study reveals generally positive interactions. Fathers who were generally responsive to their children had children with high scores in sociality and communication. A number of factors affected the quality of father interactions with children, including age, demographics, and the quality of the father's relationship with the child's mother.

What are the child and mother outcomes associated with father involvement? There is evidence that fathers can play an instrumental role in children's development (Fagan, 2000; Nord & West, 2001; Tamis-LeMonda et al., 2004), but details about critical processes are lacking. In a low-income population, it may be particularly important to know how and under what conditions fathers contribute to positive child development. Vogel et al. ("Relations Between Father Connectedness and Child Outcomes") address this with an article in the Special Issue about father presence using data provided by mothers. Results show that level and quality of presence may matter in terms of child well-being but that relations tend to vary as a function of ethnicity. Findings were generally less powerful and consistent in African American and Latin American families (compared to European Americans), indicative of the need to further explore how cultural variations and the ecological niche affect these patterns of relations. "Is One Good Parent Good Enough? Patterns of Mother and Father Parenting and Child Cognitive Outcomes at 24 and 36 Months" by Ryan, Martin, and Brooks-Gunn (this Special Issue) explores similar terrain but draws on videotaped data of mother – child and father – child interactions. The researchers found that parenting behavior is organized similarly for mothers and fathers. Their findings indicate that, when either parent acts positively in relation to the child, it has the effect of promoting adaptive functioning. A particularly significant finding from this study is that it does not seem to matter which parent acts negatively toward the child. Negative parenting has deleterious consequences. Their findings suggest that what fathers do matters; it complements what mothers do.

How can a publicly funded intervention program successfully involve fathers in program activities and in parenting? Intervention programs that target the development of infants and toddlers have traditionally focused on babies and mothers. Research on engaging fathers in such programs is limited. "Two Studies of Father Involvement in Early Head Start Programs: A National Survey and a Demonstration Program Evaluation," in this Special Issue by Raikes and Bellotti, provides information about fathers' involvement in Early Head Start programs. Findings suggest that it is not easy to productively engage fathers and that social programs aimed at supporting families may need to consider additional strategies to make programs more attractive to and supportive of fathers. (See McAllister et al., 2004; Raikes, et al., 2005; and Summers et al., 1999, for related research.)

How do cultural, regional, and community variations affect fathering and the fathers' involvement in Early Head Start? The Early Head Start research sites were selected to reflect the diversity in cultural, regional, and community variation that typifies Early Head Start. Thus, it was possible to study subgroups of fathers (specifically, African Americans, Latin Americans [including non-English-speaking Latin Americans], and European Americans) as well as to study other aspects of community context. "Exposure of Low-Income Families and Their Children to Neighborhood Violence and Paternal Antisocial Behavior," by Fitzgerald et al. (this issue), targets the issue of community violence as a factor that reduces the level and quality of paternal behavior. The authors specifically explore how both community violence and paternal antisocial behavior may be implicated in parenting practice and child well-being. They found that the combination of community violence and paternal antisocial behavior had significant negative impacts on children's emotional and cognitive functioning.

ROADMAP TO THE SPECIAL ISSUE

Authors of the articles in this Special Issue were instructed to rely on this introductory manuscript as the source of the overarching methodological details related to the Early Head Start Research and Evaluation Project data collection and the sample. Each article in this Special Issue includes a description of the subsample used in the particular study being described (for example, biological fathers or resident fathers) and may include additional information on the measures used. Two reports are exceptions to this general approach in presenting findings from the Fathers Study component of the Early Head Start national evaluation. One study represented in this Special Issue draws on data that were largely gathered at a single site

(Shannon et al., this issue), and a second study on data that were largely collected from sites other than those that participated in the Early Head Start national evaluation study (Raikes & Bellotti, this issue). Accordingly, the samples and measures used for those reports are contained within the reports themselves.

AFFILIATIONS AND ADDRESSES

Kimberly Boller, Mathematica Policy Research, Inc., 600 Alexander Park, Princeton, NJ 08543. E-mail: kboller@mathematica-mpr.com. Robert Bradley is at the University of Arkansas at Little Rock. Natasha Cabrera is at the University of Maryland. Helen H. Raikes is at the University of Nebraska–Lincoln. Barbara Pan is at Harvard University. Jeffrey Shears is at Colorado State University. Lori Roggman is at Utah State University.

ACKNOWLEDGMENTS

This article is based on work funded at least in part with Federal funds from the U.S. Department of Health and Human Services. Specifically, the work described in this article and in other articles included in this Special Issue was conducted as part of the National Early Head Start Research and Evaluation Project funded by the ACF, U.S. Department of Health and Human Services, under contract 105–95–1936 to Mathematica Policy Research, Princeton, NJ, and Columbia University's National Center for Children and Families, Teachers College, in conjunction with the Early Head Start Research Consortium. The Consortium consists of representatives from 17 programs participating in the evaluation, 15 local research teams, the evaluation contractors, and ACF. Research institutions in the Consortium (and principal researchers for conducting the research through 36 months of age) include ACF (Rachel Chazan Cohen, Judith Jerald, Esther Kresh, Helen H. Raikes, and Louisa Tarullo); Catholic University of America (Michaela Farber, Harriet Liebow, Nancy Taylor, Elizabeth Timberlake, and Shavaun Wall); Columbia University (Lisa Berlin, Christy Brady-Smith, Jeanne Brooks-Gunn, and Allison Sidle Fuligni); Harvard University (Catherine Ayoub, Barbara Alexander Pan, and Catherine Snow); Iowa State University (Dee Draper, Gayle Luze, Susan McBride, and Carla Peterson); Mathematica Policy Research (Kimberly Boller, Jill Constantine, Ellen Eliason Kisker, John M. Love, Diane Paulsell, Christine Ross, Peter Schochet, Cheri Vogel, and Welmoet van Kammen);

Medical University of South Carolina (Richard Faldowski, Gui-Young Hong, and Susan Pickrel); Michigan State University (Hiram Fitzgerald, Tom Reischl, and Rachel Schiffman); New York University (Mark Spellmann and Catherine Tamis-LeMonda); University of Arkansas (Robert Bradley, Richard Clubb, Andrea Hart, Mark Swanson, and Leanne Whiteside-Mansell); University of California, Los Angeles (Carollee Howes and Claire Hamilton); University of Colorado Health Sciences Center (Robert Emde, Jon Korfmacher, JoAnn Robinson, Paul Spicer, and Norman Watt); University of Kansas (Jane Atwater, Judith Carta, and Jean Ann Summers); University of Missouri – Columbia (Mark Fine, Jean Ispa, and Kathy Thornburg); University of Pittsburgh (Beth Green, Carol McAllister, and Robert McCall); University of Washington School of Education (Eduardo Armijo and Joseph Stowitschek); University of Washington School of Nursing (Kathryn Barnard and Susan Spieker); and Utah State University (Lisa Boyce, Gina Cook, Catherine Callow-Heusser, and Lori Roggman).

The authors thank the Consortium members who reviewed and commented on an earlier draft of this article, members of the Early Head Start Consortium Father Working Group, and editing and production staff at Mathematica. The content of this publication does not necessarily reflect the views or policies of the U.S. Department of Health and Human Services, and mention of trade names, commercial products, or organizations does not imply endorsement by the U.S. government.

REFERENCES

Administration for Children and Families. (2002a). *Making a difference in the lives of infants and toddlers and their families: The impact of Early Head Start. Volume I: Final technical report.* Washington, DC: Department of Health and Human Services.

Administration for Children and Families. (2002b). *Making a difference in the lives of infants and toddlers and their families: The impact of Early Head Start. Volume II: Final technical report appendixes.* Washington, DC: Department of Health and Human Services.

Administration for Children and Families. (2002c). *Pathways to quality and full implementation in Early Head Start programs.* Washington, DC: Department of Health and Human Services.

Administration for Children and Families. (2004a). *Health and disabilities in Early Head Start: Are families getting needed health care services?* Washington, DC: Department of Health and Human Services.

Administration for Children and Families. (2004b). *The role of Early Head Start programs in addressing the child care needs of low-income families with infants and toddlers: Influences on child care use and quality.* Washington, DC: Department of Health and Human Services.

Administration on Children, Youth and Families. (1999). *Leading the way: Characteristics and early experiences of selected Early Head Start programs. Volume I: Cross site perspectives.* Washington, DC: Department of Health and Human Services.

Administration on Children, Youth and Families. (2000). *Leading the way: Characteristics and early experiences of selected Early Head Start programs. Volume III: Program implementation.* Washington, DC: Department of Health and Human Services.

Administration on Children, Youth and Families. (2001). *Building their futures: How Early Head Start programs are changing the lives of infants and toddlers in low-income families. Volume 1: Technical report.* Washington, DC: Department of Health and Human Services.

Amato, P. (1993). Children's adjustment to divorce: Theories, hypotheses, and empirical support. *Journal of Marriage and the Family, 55,* 23–38.

Cabrera, N., Brooks-Gunn, J., Moore, K., West, J., Boller, K., & Tamis-Lemonda, C. (2002). Bridging research and policy: Including fathers of young children in national studies. In C. S. Tamis-LeMonda & N. Cabrera (Eds.), *Handbook of fatherhood involvement* (pp. 33–62). Mahwah, NJ: Lawrence Erlbaum Associates, Inc.

Cabrera, N., & Evans, V. J. (2000). Wither fathers in welfare reform. *Poverty Research News, 4,* 3–5.

Cabrera, N., Moore, K., Bronte-Tinkew, J., Halle, T., West, J., Brooks-Gunn, J., et al. (2004). The DADS initiative: Measuring father involvement in large scale surveys. In R. D. Day & M. E. Lamb (Eds.), *Conceptualizing and measuring father involvement* (pp. 417–452). Mahwah, NJ: Lawrence Erlbaum Associates, Inc.

Cabrera, N., & Peters, E. (1999). Public policies and father involvement. *Marriage and Family Review, 29,* 295–31.

Cabrera, N. J., Tamis-LeMonda, C. S., Bradley, R. H., Hofferth, S., & Lamb, M. E. (2000). Fatherhood in the twenty-first century. *Child Development, 71,* 127–136.

Carlson, M., & McLanahan, S. (2002, June). *Characteristics and antecedents of involvement by young, unmarried fathers* (Working Paper No. 02–09–FF). Princeton, NJ: Center for Research on Child Wellbeing.

Carlson, M., McLanahan, S., & Brooks-Gunn, J. (2005, March). *Unmarried but not absent: Fathers' involvement with children after a nonmarital birth* (Working Paper No. 05–07–FF). Princeton, NJ: Center for Research on Child Wellbeing.

Cherlin, A. J., Furstenberg, F. F., Chase-Landsdale, P. L., Kiernan, K. E., Robins, P. K., Morrison, D. R., et al. (1991). Longitudinal studies of effects of divorce on children in Great Britain and the United States. *Science, 252,* 1386–1389.

Cherlin, A. J., & Griffin, J. (1998). Report of the working group on the methodology of studying fathers. In *Nurturing fatherhood: Improving data and research on male fertility, family formation and fatherhood* (pp. 173–206). Washington, DC: Federal Interagency Forum on Child and Family Statistics.

Clarke-Stewart, A. (1978). And daddy makes three: The father's impact on mother and young child. *Child Development, 49*(2), 466–478.

Coley, R. L. (2001). (In)visible men: Emerging research on low-income, unmarried, and minority fathers. *American Psychologist, 56,* 743–753.

Cummings, E. M., & O'Reilly, A. W. (1997). Fathers in family context: Effects of marital quality on child adjustment. In M. E. Lamb (Ed.), *The role of the father in child development* (3rd ed., pp. 49–65, 318–325). New York: Wiley.

Doherty, W. J., Kouneski, E. F., & Erikson, M. F. (1998). Responsible fathering: An overview and conceptual framework. *Journal of Marriage and the Family, 60,* 277–292.

Duncan, G. J., & Brooks-Gunn, J. (Eds.). (1997). *Consequences of growing up poor.* New York: Russell Sage Foundation.

Edin, K., & Lein, L. (1997). *Making ends meet: How single mothers survive welfare and low-wage work.* New York: Russell Sage Foundation.

Ellis, B. J., Bates, J. E., Dodge, K. A., Fergusson, D. M., Horwood, L. J., Pettit, G. S., et al. (2003). Does father absence place daughters at special risk for early sexual activity? *Child Development, 74*, 801–822.

Fagan, J. (2000). African American and Puerto Rican American parenting styles, parental involvement, and Head Start children's social competence. *Merrill-Palmer Quarterly, 46*, 592–612.

Federal Interagency Forum on Child and Family Statistics. (1998). *Nurturing fatherhood: Improving data and research on male fertility, family formation and fatherhood.* Washington DC: Federal Author.

Fincham, F. (1998). Child development and marital relations. *Child Development, 69*, 543–574.

Garfinkel, I., McLanahan, D., & Hanson, T. (1998). A patchwork portrait of nonresident fathers. In I. Garfinkel, S. McLanahan, D. Meyer, & J. Seltzer (Eds.), *Fathers under fire: The revolution in child support enforcement* (pp. 31–60). New York: Russell Sage Foundation.

Goeke-Morey, M. C., & Cummings, E. C. (2005, June). *Impact of father involvement: A closer look at indirect effects models involving attachment, marriage and child adjustment.* Paper presented at the National Fatherhood Forum, College Park, MD.

Hernandez, D., & Brandon, P. (2002). Who are the fathers of today? In C. S. Tamis-LeMonda & N. Cabrera (Eds.), *Handbook of fatherhood involvement* (pp. 33–62). Mahwah, NJ: Lawrence Erlbaum Associates, Inc.

Hetherington, E. M., & Stanley-Hagan, M. (1986). Divorced fathers: Stress, coping, and adjustment. In M. E. Lamb (Ed.), *The father's role: Applied perspectives* (pp. 103–134). New York: Wiley.

Hijjawi, G. R., Wilson, M., & Turkheimer, E. (2003, February). *An exploratory analysis of father involvement in low-income families* (Working Paper No. 03–01–FF). Princeton, NJ: Center for Research on Child Wellbeing.

Ispa, J. M., Fine, M. A., Halgunseth, L. C., Harper, S., Robinson, J., Boyce, L., et al. (2004). Maternal intrusiveness, maternal warmth, and mother–toddler relationship outcomes: Variation across low-income ethnic and acculturation groups. *Child Development, 75*, 1613–1631.

Kalil, A. (2003, October). *Fathers' perceptions of paternal roles: Variations by marital status and living arrangements* (Working Paper No. 03–12–FF). Princeton, NJ: Center for Research on Child Wellbeing.

Lamb, M. E. (1997). The development of father–infant relationships. In M. E. Lamb (Ed.), The role of the father in child development (3rd ed., pp. 104–120). New York: Wiley.

Lamb, M. E. (1999). *Parenting and child development in "nontraditional" families.* Mahwah, NJ: Lawrence Erlbaum Associates, Inc.

Lewis, C. (1997). Fathers and preschoolers. In M. E. Lamb (Ed.), *The role of the father in child development* (3rd ed., pp. 121–142). New York: Wiley.

Lewis, M., Feiring, C., & Weinraub, M. (1981). The father as a member of the child's social network. In M. E. Lamb (Ed.), *The role of the father in child development* (2nd ed., pp. 259–294). New York: Wiley.

Lewis, M., & Weinraub, M. (1976). The father's role in the child's social network. In M. E. Lamb (Ed.), *The role of the father in child development* (1st ed., pp. 157–184). New York: Plenum.

Love, J. M., Kisker, E. E., Ross, C., Raikes, H., Constantine, J., Boller, K., et al. (2005). The effectiveness of Early Head Start for 3-year-old children and their parents: Lessons for policy and programs. *Developmental Psychology, 41*(6), 885–901.

Martin, E., & Siegel, P. (1998). New directions for exploring fathers' attachment to households. In *Nurturing fatherhood: Improving data and research on male fertility, family formation and fa-*

therhood (pp. 435–441). Washington, DC: Federal Interagency Forum on Child and Family Statistics.

McAdoo, J. L. (1993). The roles of African American fathers: An ecological perspective. Families in society: *The Journal of Contemporary Human Services, 74,* 28–35.

McAllister, C. L., Wilson, P. C., & Burton, J. (2004). From sports fans to nurturers: An Early Head Start program's evolution toward father involvement. *Fathering, 2,* 31–60.

McLanahan, S., & Sandefur, S. (1994). Growing up with a single parent: What hurts, what helps. Cambridge, MA: Harvard University Press.

McLoyd, V. C. (1998). Socioeconomic disadvantage and child development. *American Psychologist, 53,* 185–204.

McLoyd, V. C., Cauce, A. M., Takeuchi, D., & Wilson, L. (2000). Marital processes and parental socialization in families of color: A decade review of research. *Journal of Marriage and the Family, 62,* 1070–1093.

Miles, M. B., & Huberman, A. M. (1994). *Qualitative data analysis: An expanded sourcebook* (2nd ed.). Thousand Oaks, CA: Sage.

Newcomer, S., & Udry, R. J. (1987). Parental marital status effects on adolescent sexual behavior. *Journal of Marriage and the Family, 49,* 235–240.

Nord, C. W., & West, J. (2001). *Fathers' and mothers' involvement in their children's schools by family type and resident status.* Washington, DC: U.S. Department of Education, National Center for Education Statistics.

Parke, R. (2002). Fathers' contributions to children's peer relations. In C. Tamis-LeMonda & N. Cabrera (Eds.), *Handbook of father involvement: Multidisciplinary perspectives* (pp. 141–168). Mahwah, NJ: Lawrence Erlbaum Associates, Inc.

Raikes, H., Roggman, L., & Summers, J. (2005). Father involvement in Early Head Start programs. *Fathering, 3,* 29–58.

Reichman, N., Teitler, J., Garfinkel, I., & McLanahan, S. (2001). The fragile families and child wellbeing study: Sample and design. *Children and Youth Services Review, 23,* 303–326.

Roggman, L. A., Fitzgerald, H. E., Bradley, R. H., & Raikes, H. (2002). Methodological, measurement, and design issues in studying fathers: An interdisciplinary perspective. In C. S. Tamis-LeMonda & N. Cabrera (Eds.), *Handbook of fatherhood involvement* (pp. 33–62). Mahwah, NJ: Lawrence Erlbaum Associates, Inc.

Shannon, J. D., Tamis-LeMonda, C. S., London, K., & Cabrera, N. (2002). Beyond rough and tumble: Low-income fathers' interactions and children's cognitive development at 24 months. *Parenting: Science and Practice, 2,* 77–104.

Sorenson, E., & Pomper, K. (2003, May). *Assessing the causal relationship between child support and visitation.* Paper presented at the annual meeting of the Population Association of America, Minneapolis, MN.

Summers, J. A., Boller, K., & Raikes, H. (2004). Preferences and perceptions about getting support expressed by low-income fathers. *Fathering, 2,* 61–82.

Summers, J. A., Spicer, P., Pan, B., Shaw, S., Lanager, M., McAllister, C., et al. (1999). *Fathers' roles and father involvement in Early Head Start programs: Report from a pilot study.* Unpublished manuscript.

Tamis-LeMonda, C. S., Shannon, J. D., Cabrera, N. J., & Lamb, M. E. (2004). Fathers and mothers at play with their 2- and 3-year-olds: Contributions to language and cognitive development. *Child Development, 75,* 1806–1820.

Thompson, R. A. (1986). Fathers and the child's best interests: Judicial decision-making in custody disputes. In M. E. Lamb (Ed.), *The father's role: Applied perspectives* (pp. 61–102). New York: Wiley.

U.S. Department of Health and Human Services. (1994). *The statement of the Advisory Committee on Services for Families with Infants and Toddlers* (Department of Health and Human Services Publication No. 615–032/03062). Washington, DC: Department of Health and Human Services.

Western, B., & McLanahan, S. (2000). Fathers behind bars: The impact of incarceration on family formation. In G. L. Fox & M. L. Benson (Eds.), *Families, crime, and criminal justice: Vol. 2. Charting the linkages* (pp. 307–322). New York: JAI.

Wilson, M., & Brooks-Gunn, J. (2001, January). *The health status and behaviors of unwed fathers* (Working Paper No. 01–01–FF). Princeton, NJ: Center for Research on Child Wellbeing.

PARENTING: SCIENCE AND PRACTICE
April–September 2006 Volume 6 Numbers 2 & 3 Pages 145–165

The Meaning of "Good Fatherhood:" Low-Income Fathers' Social Constructions of Their Roles

Jean Ann Summers, Kimberly Boller,
Rachel F. Schiffman, and Helen H. Raikes

SYNOPSIS

Objective. To gain a better understanding of how low-income fathers of young children think about their role as fathers, we conducted a qualitative inquiry into the beliefs of fathers of 24-month-old children about what "good fatherhood" means to them. ***Design.*** The 575 open-ended interviews, collected in 14 Early Head Start Fathers of Toddlers Qualitative Interview Substudy sites around the United States were analyzed using NUD*IST qualitative software to code and categorize the various roles fathers identified as important to them and their children. ***Results.*** Four broad types of roles were identified: (1) providing a stable environment (e.g., providing a living, "being there" emotionally and physically), (2) teaching (e.g., giving guidance, exposing their child to the world), (3) physical interaction (e.g., play, caregiving), and (4) emotional support (e.g., providing love, building self-esteem). ***Conclusion.*** The beliefs of these men are considered in the context of historical perceptions of fatherhood, as well as their implications for generative theories of fatherhood. Overall, fathers articulated a strong sense of commitment and intentionality in their plans for interactions with their children. Our findings provide opportunities for service providers and policymakers to develop positive strategies to ensure fathers' ability to carry out their intentions.

INTRODUCTION

Recent approaches to fatherhood research have proposed a generative perspective that recommends studying the activities fathers do for their children through a sense of responsible caring (Hawkins & Dollahite, 1997). The generative perspective moves beyond the "deficit paradigm" of research that focused on the effects of father absence rather than on the positive and complex roles fathers often play (Marsiglio, Amato, Day, & Lamb, 2000). A "generative perspective" presents an image, informed by the values of a culture, about just how a "good father" should act.

Lamb, Pleck, Charnov, and Levine (1987) articulated a framework for understanding positive father involvement that includes fathers' engagement, accessibility, and responsibility toward their children. Another framework for understanding father involvement is the "social capital" view, in which fathers influence children through direct interactions with them, indirect connections facilitated for children through fathers' resources, and the involvement by fathers with the community groups and institutions in which children participate (Marsiglio, Amato, Day, & Lamb, 2000). Still another framework for generative fathering is the sociohistorical point of view, analyzing how father roles have changed over time. In American culture, for example, the definition of "good father" has shifted over time from a more traditional view that mothers and fathers occupy discretely different roles (with fathers in primarily a provider role) to the recent view that mothers and fathers are coparents, sharing all parenting roles (E. H. Pleck & Pleck, 1997). These generative formulations attribute to fathers a sense of responsible caring, a desire to care for and meet their child's needs (Hawkins & Dollahite, 1997). The assumption of positive intent is the basis for studies of fatherhood focusing on understanding how men perceive and construct their identities as fathers (Marsiglio et al., 2000).

Although the popular culture has embraced the idea of fathers as a highly visible and positive force in all aspects of their children's lives, the image of low-income fathers remains more nebulous and negative. Assumptions about low-income fathers encompass expectations of absence and neglect, resulting in stereotypes about "deadbeat dads" that became codified in welfare reform legislation focused on strengthening child support enforcement (Child Support Performance and Incentive Act of 1998). More recent studies suggest that low-income and nonresident or minority fathers are in fact more involved with their children than previously thought (Cabrera et al., 2004; Salem, Zimmerman, & Notaro, 1998).

A conceptual framework for "responsible fathering" proposed by Doherty, Kouneski, and Erickson (1998) may contribute to our understanding of how low-income fathers might differ from middle-income fathers. Doherty and colleagues noted that mother's levels of engagement, accessibility, and responsibility toward their child may tend to remain uniformly high regardless of various influences in their lives. In contrast, they argue that father involvement may be strongly influenced by a number of contextual features of the relationships, environment, and culture surrounding them. More specifically, in their model, the father's ability to achieve his vision of a "good father" may be influenced by (1) his own knowledge, skills, commitment, and experiences with his own father; (2) his relationship with his child's mother; (3) the mother's attitudes and expectations toward the father; (4) contextual factors such as employment, economic factors, and cultural expectations; and (5) child factors such as behavioral challenges, gender, and age.

Support for a large part of the Doherty et al. (1998) model is available in the literature. With respect to the coparenting relationship, for example, Allen and Hawkins (1999) found that maternal "gatekeeping" inhibited greater father involvement in family work. McBride and Rane (1998) also found that the mothers' support and a shared parenting philosophy were significant predictors for father involvement with their children. With respect to contextual and cultural factors, studies suggest that fathers with high levels of overtime in their work had less positive relationships with their sons and daughters (Crouter, Bumpus, Head, & McHale, 2001). Furthermore, low-income fathers who perceive themselves as less than adequate providers tend to have reduced or negative interactions with their children (Harold-Goldsmith, Radin, & Eccles, 1988; Jones, 1991; LaRossa & Reitzes, 1993). Finally, with respect to child characteristics, McBride, Schoppe, and Rane (2002) found more significant associations between child temperament and involvement for fathers than for mothers.

Less well explored in this framework, especially for low-income or minority fathers, is the first component of the Doherty model — the father's own sense of his role, encompassing his own knowledge, commitment, and understanding of what he should be doing. Without knowing the initial intent that fathers bring to their role, there seems to be very little point in exploring the various environmental, partner relationship, and child characteristics that may or may not bend the trajectory of that intent. Even more, without knowing what low-income men think about fathering, policymakers and service providers are designing supports and setting policies in a vacuum.

This study focuses a generative lens on the question of how low-income men perceive their role as fathers. Specifically, we ask the following: What is the understanding of fathers from low-income backgrounds of the meaning of "good fatherhood?" Because of the exploratory nature of this question, we considered a qualitative approach to be the most appropriate paradigm.

METHODS

Sample

This study utilizes data from the embedded qualitative interviews conducted as part of the Fathers of Toddlers Qualitative Interview Substudy when children were 24 months old. The overall design and approach are described in the introductory article for this Special Issue (see Boller et al., this issue). The qualitative portions of the interview were audiotaped. Accounting for tapes which were inaudible or defective, the total sample size for the qualitative analysis was 575 fathers or father figures. Forty-nine percent were from the Early Head Start group, and 51% were from the control group. On average, 41 fathers from each of the 14 sites participated in the study on fathers; 66% were resident, biological fathers; 16% were nonresident, biological fathers; 15% were resident father figures (such as the mother's husband or partner or the child's grandfather); and 4% were nonresident father figures (with rounding, the total is greater than 100%). The fathers' characteristics at the time of the interview are shown in the demographic tables provided in the methodological description in Boller et al. (this issue). Compared with the sample of nonrespondents, more of the fathers who participated in the Father Study were resident biological fathers, and more were married to their child's mother (Cabrera et al., 2004).

Interview Protocol and Procedure

The qualitative interview protocol for the 24-month interview included six primary or "grand tour" (Miles & Huberman, 1994) questions: (1) What does being a "good father" mean to you? (2) How has becoming a father impacted your life? (3) Talk about your experiences with your own father. (4) What kinds of help or support do you get to do your job as a father? (5) What gets in the way of being a father? (6) What are you proudest of about your child? For each grand tour question, the Father Studies Work Group developed a series of suggested probes to serve as guidelines for the interviewers. The probes were intended to elicit more elaborative responses to these questions. This report addresses the first research question.

The interviewers in the 14 Early Head Start Father Study sites were approximately evenly divided between men and women. All interviewers were given a manual and a demonstration videotape to provide training in techniques of qualitative interviewing. The national coordinator of the qualitative component of the father interview held three conference calls during the early stages of data collection for the 24-month interview to provide guidance, feedback, and peer-debriefing about early results to the interviewers, facilitate discussion, and generate additional probes that might be helpful. The qualitative interview questions were interspersed in three different places throughout the quantitative protocol; interviewers turned the tape recorders on only for these qualitative questions. The taped portions of the interviews averaged about 20 min.

Data Analysis

Audiotapes of the interviews were transcribed; Spanish language interviews (15% of the total sample) were transcribed in Spanish and translated to English. The researchers at each site received copies of all their transcripts and were asked to provide an assessment of the accuracy of a randomly selected set of the transcripts. Two sites (New York and Vermont) conducted accuracy checks of samples of their transcripts by listening to the tapes while following the transcripts, and reported no substantive corrections to transcript content as a result of this accuracy check.

An initial framework for analysis (Miles & Huberman, 1994) used the results of a pilot study involving focus groups conducted in four of the Early Head Start Father Workgroup sites (see Summers et al., 1999). This framework formed the basis for an initial "Index Tree" and coding "nodes" in the NUD*IST qualitative software program. The first author and two research assistants (the Analysis Team) completed the coding process by comparing each successive transcript with the coding structure and adding or modifying the codes based on the new material. This process is called the constant comparison method (Anfara, Brown, & Mangione, 2002). After coding the first 234 transcripts, the Analysis Team examined the codes and their definitions as a team and revised the analytical framework and coding structure. A randomly selected sample of 10% of reports from the coded categories were reviewed to determine whether the text had been appropriately coded. Text units on which Analysis Team members disagreed were discussed and either retained with a revision or clarification of the code, or reassigned to a different code. The Father Studies Work Group as a whole also reviewed the revised coding structure and provided conceptual feedback. In addition, one site (Michigan) independently coded transcripts from their site using the revised structure, and reported general agreement with the appropriateness of the codes. This code – recode strategy is a method in qualitative methodology for establishing "dependability," a concept analogous to reliability in quantitative research; because it is a consensus-building process resulting in revisions of both the codes and the coding assigned to individual narrative passages, no statistical measures of reliability are appropriate (Anfara et al., 2002).

The initial 234 transcripts were recoded using the revised coding structure, and the remaining transcripts from the 24-month father interviews were then coded. This report presents the data reflecting a total of 575 transcripts of from the open-ended interviews from the 24-month data collection. The qualitative coders were "blind" to the demographic characteristics of respondents, because the primary purpose was to provide an inventory of the range and types of roles these men believe fathers should have. Therefore, the quotations presented later do not specify either the site or any demographic characteristics of the respondent quoted.

RESULTS

The themes identified from this analysis suggest that these fathers talked of their roles in terms of how they saw themselves benefiting their children: (1) as a source of stability — "being there," providing support; (2) as a mentor and teacher — guiding, shaping values, teaching children; (3) as a caregiver — engaging in physical interactions, providing care; and (4) as a nurturer — providing emotional support and love. Table 1 provides definitions of these categories and subcategories. The order in which these subcategories is presented is not indicative of their relative importance or salience to the fathers. Rather, they represent the order in which the themes emerged as the coders went through transcripts one after the other using the constant comparison method. The themes should be considered equally important from the respondents' perspectives, in part because an approximately equal number of fathers spoke of each of the main categories and in part because the respondents were not asked to prioritize or otherwise choose the "most" important roles for fathers. It was typical for a section of a transcript to receive codes from at least two, and often many, of the subcategories within the four broad themes. Many fathers responded to this question by reeling off an extensive list of roles, for example:

> Making sure that there is food on the table for my child. Of course, a roof over her head. Provide her with any kind of knowledge from me. If she has any questions ... Being there when they need you, helping them when they get hurt, playing with them, having a good time with them, just showing them you're part of their life, and they can always be dependent on you to be there for them.

In short, these respondents appeared to see their roles as multifaceted. The following sections consider the meaning of each of the four broad themes in greater detail.

"Being There" — Bedrock of Support

This category refers to fathers' conceptualizations of themselves as a kind of "bedrock" of support for their children. That support manifests in several forms, including actual and spiritual presence, making sure the family is financially secure and safe from harm, and making sure the fam-

TABLE 1

Roles of a "Good Father" Identified by Fathers of Low-Income Families

Category Definition	Subcategory Definitions
I. Stability: Fathers describe the importance of promoting a secure and stable environment for their children.	I.A. "Be There:" Fathers describe the importance of being generally available to their children, both physically and emotionally, for consistent periods of time. I.B. Protection: Fathers describe their role as providing physical and emotional protection and security to their children. I.C. Partnership: Fathers describe the importance of a functional partnership with their child's mother, or having both parents present in the child's life. I.D. Financial: Fathers describe the importance of providing financial support to their children.
II. Teaching: Fathers describe their role as one of teacher, guide, or disciplinarian for their children.	II.A. General Teaching, Discipline: Fathers describe their role as generally teaching "right from wrong," providing discipline, guiding the child. II.B. Teaching Content: Fathers address specific content they wish to teach their children, for example, academics, values, religion, gender differences. II.C. Teaching Methods: Fathers express an opinion about the appropriate methods fathers should employ to teach their children, for example, being consistent, role modeling, answering child's questions, etc.
III. Physical Interaction: Fathers describe the importance of physical involvement with their children.	III.A. Caregiving: Fathers describe engaging in daily caregiving chores, including "babysitting," feeding, etc. III.B. Play and Recreation: Fathers describe physical gross motor play or playing with toys, etc. III.C. Spend Time, Outings: Fathers describe the importance of simply "spending time" with their children, or emphasize taking children with them on outings or to events.
IV. Emotional: Fathers describe the importance of providing emotional care and support for their children.	IV.A. Love: Fathers refer to the importance of demonstrating love for their children. IV.B. Communication: Fathers describe the importance of having positive communication with their children. IV.C. Support: Fathers describe the importance of building their child's self-esteem and otherwise being emotionally supportive. IV.D. Cuddling, Comfort: Fathers describe rocking, cuddling, or comforting their children.

ily works as a unit. Thus, the four subcategories within this broad theme included the following: (1) providing financial support, (2) "being there," (3) forming a stable partnership with the child's mother, and (4) providing protection.

Financial support. Some fathers referred to financial support as a hallmark of a "good father." This meant "putting food on the table," "making sure they have what they need," or even "providing some of those extras." As one father said, "whenever I'm lacking work I get worried because I think about my children. They have to be dressed and fed, ... and if I didn't work I don't know what would happen." Commentary about financial support was not as strongly emphasized in many of the transcripts. One possible interpretation is that these fathers were responding to the question about what it meant to be a good father; perhaps, financial support was a minimum requirement, and being a good father went beyond that. For example, the comments of one father were typical of a number of similar responses that led us to this interpretation:

> I think you need everything to raise a son: You need the financial capability of raising a son and you need the love. Some people try to do one and not the other. They think since they're paying child support that they are doing their job as a father, or they just spend time with their [child] and think they're doing their job as a father. I think you need to do both.

Be there. The phrase "being there" (or "be there") was used often. Interviewers routinely asked the respondent to elaborate about this term. A typical response was "no matter what the circumstances are, you're always there for them." The overall sense was that "being there" meant being present in a child's life and also accessible, both physically and emotionally. We placed the concept of "being there" within the broader theme of stability because it was used often in the context of a father's resolve to be a consistent and reliable source of support to the child: "Being there when they need you, helping them when they get hurt." Or, in good times, "being there" meant providing encouragement and witnessing accomplishments. See the following, for example:

> I didn't have anybody to be there for me as a father ... And as far as my mom, she went through a rocky period where she had to work 2 or 3 jobs ... . Like, even through high school, mom was at one wrestling tournament the entire time. I did quite well, and yet I didn't

> have anyone there to say wow, you did that. ... I'd like to make sure that [my kids] know that. That's being there.

Partnership with the child's mother. Some fathers addressed the concept that a "good" father provided a stable environment for his children by establishing a stable relationship with their mother. These respondents were often referring to trends about single parenting or fatherless households, for example:

> I know that's an important part of every child of having their father there. A mother can't just raise a child, it takes two parents. And the combination of the both .... I mean we as Afro-Americans, we have a lot of single parents out here. And it's important that these families get back together.

Partnership with the mother also referred to the need for parents to work together to send consistent messages to their children, to pitch in together and support one another's efforts:

> [It's] about having patience, sometimes it's difficult. That's where the mother comes in, you have to play off each other .... Some days one of you is not going to have the patience and that's where the other one can step up, and that's just very important.

Protection. Some respondents also referred to the father's role as a protector — for example, "make sure that I protect my family from anything that might happen to them." Fathers considered it important for their children to see them as a source of protection and security: "She knows I'm always here to protect her. Yesterday her uncle was shooting off poppers, and she's afraid of loud noises, and so she comes running to me 'cause I'm her daddy." Respondents talked about making sure the child avoided such dangers as electrical outlets or traffic. Others spoke in more general terms about protecting children from the bad influences of media or peer groups, or simply providing a sense of security for the child: "They're young right now and they're real vulnerable to everything, so you've got to be real strong for them."

Teaching, Guiding, "Raising" the Child

Over and over, teaching and role modeling, raising and shaping a child, emerged as a very central part of their role in the minds of these fathers. Fathers emphasized their responsibilities to expose children to the world, to help them learn social values, and to gain an education. Respondents discussed the importance of the father's role as the disciplinarian, teacher, or authority figure for children. These discussions included specific comments describing the content or types of things they wanted to teach (e.g., education, social values), as well as the teaching methods or strategies to be used in teaching. The following is how one father put it when asked what surprised him about becoming a father:

> It's harder than I thought ... . The providing isn't the hard part. It's the everyday — you gotta set an example for them, you gotta teach them, you worry you don't teach them enough, you don't teach them what they need. That's the part that's more difficult than I thought it would be.

The subcategories related to teaching included both content (i.e., what fathers hoped to teach) and process (i.e., how fathers proposed to teach). These include the following: (1) teaching values for life, teaching specific content (e.g., academics, attitudes); and (2) teaching methods (e.g., role modeling, having conversations).

Teaching, developing values for life. A pervasive phrase was the fathers' perceived responsibility to teach their children "right from wrong." This phrase, like "being there," had broad meaning — it referred to providing structure, authority, self-discipline, and a moral sense of how to act and treat others. One father said the following:

> Probably fathers help set up more of our conscience as an early kid, you know, in your early development. Like what's right and what's wrong, what's unsafe and what's safe, and that kind of stuff. And I think that's probably where being there all the time kind of really provides a benefit.

Teaching content. Many fathers expressed a clear idea about the kinds of things they wanted their children to learn. Often their purpose was to teach social values and to prepare the young child for the pitfalls of the teen years, such as gangs or drugs. See the following, for example:

> Being a good father means I'm taking the time to spend quality time with my children, help them learn good manners, to be polite, how to play with each other, be polite to adults. Get them well-grounded in morals early so when they grow up they won't have problems; go through the teen years with those problems ... . So they learn that early and they know what to expect [from life] later on.

Fathers also talked of instilling values such as a work ethic or self-reliance, providing spiritual or religious guidance, and teaching gender expectations ("what it is to be a man"). These respondents also expressed a need to emphasize education with their children. Many spoke of a strong desire to make sure their children go farther in school than they did, or to make sure children realize that getting an education is a key to their future well-being: "Basically, try to provide them with a good education, make them understand how to see it through, and why they should, make them understand that. Pretty much, if you are going to accomplish that, and feed them, too, you've provided for them."

Teaching methods. Respondents also discussed the strategies they should use to teach their children. Fathers described drilling or playing games to teach children their letters or numbers, to tie shoes, and so on. With respect to discipline, some fathers noted the importance of consistency and fairness. Others spoke of being ready and willing to answer children's questions, to provide information and advice. Still other fathers talked about being involved in their child's activities:

> Like if [child] wants to play in a band, we need to get her the instrument and lessons she needs, help her out any way we can. Go to her concerts. If she wants to play on the girl's basketball team, go out and shoot some baskets with her. Make sure we go to the games .... do everything possible to support her.

Far more pervasive however, was the idea that fathers should teach by serving as a role model. The terms *role model, positive role model, being a good example,* or being *someone to look up to* were used frequently. Many responded to the question about the impact of fatherhood on their lives by saying they had curtailed their "bad habits" or otherwise changed their lives to "set a good example." As one father put it bluntly, "to be a good father one has to be a good man." Fathers spoke of being a role model by pursuing their education, by holding down jobs, by avoiding drugs and violence, and so on. One stepfather described at length the importance of being a role model:

> I always try to be a positive role model .... I think it's important for her to have that male role model because her biological dad is choosing not to be a part of what's going on .... I know a lot of things I do she looks up to. So, if I have that expectation of her I have to do the same thing myself.

Physical Interactions and Caregiving

Comments about physical interactions and caregiving (family activities) described a broad range of direct exchanges with children, including (1) simply spending time with children, (2) serving as a general caregiver (e.g., feeding, diapering), and (3) playing with their children.

Spending time. Comments about "spending time" included simply "hanging out" with their children or taking them along on outings. These fathers responded to the question, "What are some of the things you do that make you feel you are a good father?" by describing the inclusion of their children in their daily routines, such as taking them along on errands, or allowing them to "help" with chores or repairs.: "He's my little buddy. We do everything together." Others described more child-focused "spending time" activities, such as taking the child to the park, playing with the child in the backyard, or reading or watching television. Many of these respondents appeared to be mindful of the purpose of the activity: "Showing them how to do things right ... Let them experience things. Pretty much just let them get to know what they're getting into when they're getting into life." In other words, many of these fathers appeared to be aware of the teaching or shaping implications of even casual interactions with their children.

General caregiving. Fathers talked of "taking care of" their children, which included feeding, diapering, bathing, and putting the child to bed:

> For the past year, I have been the one that's got [child] up. [Wife] has to leave for work early in the morning, and so I get [child] up and feed her, do her hair, things like that, and get her off to preschool while I go to school and work, and that's been fun. I've definitely gotten better at it.

As this quote suggests, comments about caregiving were often made in the context of describing the division of responsibilities with the child's mother (e.g., "I take care of her when mom can't."). Some couples solved their child care needs by working opposite shifts, so that one would be home with the children at all times: "When I'm working [wife] will clean the house and feed her lunch. When I get home I read to her, I give her a bath and put her to bed ... The split is that [wife] pretty much does everything when I'm not here, and when I'm home it's the opposite."

Physical play and recreation. Many fathers talked about playing with their children. A typical response to this question, "What are some of the things that you do that make you feel like you're being a good father?" was as follows:

> I play with them … . When they smile and they're happy as can be, you can tell it on their face. I've always grown believing you should really play with children. Enjoy them while they're around 'cause they're gone really before you know it.

Play seemed to be a special purview of fathers: "She's probably more mommy's when she's sick and she likes to play with daddy. I'll get down on my knees and chase her around; act like I'm going to get her."

Emotional Support

The love of these men for their children was palpable. Especially when asked about the impact of becoming a father on their lives, these men talked of being overwhelmed with feelings of love that they had not anticipated. An often-used term was *joy*. Many fathers described the "warm and fuzzy" feelings they felt when their child displayed excited happiness to see them: "To hear him say 'daddy, daddy, daddy!' There's nothing like it." "Every time I pick him up from school … I see his face and he calls me daddy and starts running to me. That makes me happy." Another father described his daughter's reactions when he came home from work:

> Well, I think it is just pure joy. I mean when I come home at night, she's there with a big smile and wants me—well, we call it uppy—it means pick her up. And she wants to be picked up and hugged. And I give her a hug and squeeze and ask her how the day was. It's just a joy having her around.

It is not surprising that fathers who felt their child had brought so much love into their life also emphasized giving back a strong sense of love and emotional support. Many of these men described their own fathers as emotionally distant and talked about wanting to be more emotionally available with their own children. Some of these men talked of being abused or abandoned by their fathers, but others simply described their fathers as "too busy" or unable to express feelings. One father put it this way:

I: Talk about your experiences with your father when you were a child. What was he like? Was there something you wish had been different?

R: Yes, many things. That he would love us because he has never shown that he loved us. He was always gone, traveling I don't know where. I would have liked him to be the way I am with my children. Love them, hug them, kiss them, take them places and he never went anywhere with us. Never showed, well maybe he did love us, but he never showed it and that is why I want to be different from him, not like him. Maybe in his heart he did love us, but we never got a hug from him, not a kiss, never took us out on a weekend. We never knew any such thing and that's why I'm telling you I'm different with my children, the opposite.

General discussions of providing emotional support included fathers' descriptions of their role as making a child feel loved, or encouraging children and developing self-esteem, and the strategies for providing emotional support included, for some fathers, anticipating an open communication with one's child, and for others — focusing more on their child's current age — rocking, cuddling, or comforting their child.

Love. Some fathers described the importance of "giving all the love that one can" to their children. Being a good father means the following: "Showing them each and every day that you care about them, that they are loved, that they mean the world to you and that they would be really, really missed if they were ever lost." A few fathers thought that establishing love between a father and child required more conscious effort than the mother - child bond:

> With the mother maybe there is more of an immediate bond ... but as a man, it's more in the experiences ... sometimes I'll take her on my chest and she'll lean up and her eyes look at me, and I start talking to her and that kind of stuff, like she kind of understands me, so that's the bonding.

Encouragement. A variety of comments concerned the importance of making a child feel wanted and praising a child for his or her accomplishments: "You've got to let them know that when they achieve you really appreciate it, and encourage it more. Because if you don't care, then the kid ain't going to care." Building a child's self-esteem also included treating a child with dignity and respect: "relating to them, talking to them one-on-one, rather than talking to them as a dog or an object, eye-to-eye, person-to-person."

Communication. Some respondents emphasized establishing good communication with their children. Most of these comments focused on the relationship fathers hoped to develop as their children grew older: "The main thing is to make sure that you're able to talk and communicate with your kids, that you have some kind of open line of communication with them." For some, communication once again had a teaching function, in that fathers talked of letting their children know their opinions about life, to understand their life experiences, and ideas of how to be successful in the world:

> If he can hear me say the things I've learned ... not hammer it into him like I'm grilling him or quizzing him, but just this is my experiences, this is what I believe and why I believe it, and this is the way the world works according to me. They can believe what they want and learn the rest for themselves. When they are faced with situations they might hear my voice in their head.

A common theme about communication was fathers' concern that their children should "feel free" to talk with them, "not be afraid" to come to them with questions or issues:

> I want to be connected with my kids, not to where when they get older they're scared to talk to me. I want to be able to express everything but still be there for them and not hide things from me or feel that there's no way I should be right there with them.

Touching, holding, and comforting. A few fathers described the importance of fathers comforting, cuddling, rocking, or otherwise physically touching their children: "Take your time. Instead of walking by your kid, take your time and pat him on the head and pick him up." Comforting a child who is hurt or ill was considered an important part of fathering by these respondents, and one that they found rewarding:

> Like when she wakes up in the middle [of the night] and calls out for daddy. So I'll ... just go on and get her you know, like comfort her, get her quiet and stuff, and she'll go on back to sleep and make me feel good.

DISCUSSION

Before considering the implications of this study, we should note its limitations. From the perspective of qualitative methodology, the transcripts analyzed here do not present the kind of prolonged engagement and contextual - environmental context to allow in-depth exploration of how these fathers arrived at their perspectives. And these data do not give us an idea of how these concepts of fatherhood play out in their daily life and actual behavior. Also, the primary purpose of this study was to determine the broad range of father perspectives about their role; the qualitative team was blind to the differing demographic characteristics of the men represented in these transcripts. Therefore, we cannot draw conclusions about variations in these perspectives to trace the cultural or demographic roots of those possible differences. Finally, the fathers included in this study were accessed through the mothers of their children and consisted, therefore, primarily of men who had positive or at least neutral relationships with their partners. Therefore, we likely have a somewhat rosier view of father perspectives than may be the case for low-income fathers more generally. With these caveats in mind, we may draw some tentative conclusions and implications.

The voices of these low-income men present evidence that they have a clear image of a "good father." Collectively, a reading across all the transcripts presents a vision with multiple dimensions encompassing a range of roles from provider to nurturer to teacher. The roles they identify are expressed in terms of popular images and social icons about fathers and fathering that are deeply embedded in the culture. They confirm the range of traditional (e.g., providing and protecting, teaching) and recent "coparenting" (e.g., caregiving, providing emotional support) identified by E. H. Pleck and Pleck (1997). However, instead of dropping the more traditional roles, these fathers appear to embrace them all. In other words, rather than an evolution from one view of parenthood to another, these fathers appear to be acquiring new roles without rejecting or modifying the old ones.

Likewise, these low-income fathers reflect the concept of the "involved" father as defined by Lamb and his colleagues (1987). Their comments include descriptions of engagement (through play, physical caregiving, taking the child with them on outings), accessibility (by "spending time," "being there," and otherwise emphasizing their physical and emotional presence), and responsibility (by providing material support and creating a stable family life). Finally, each of the four themes emerging in this study sheds light on low-income fathers' sense of commitment and intentionality, which is one of the components of the framework presented by Doherty and colleagues (1998).

In these interviews, taken around the time of their child's second birthday, these respondents present a fierce determination to be a force for stability in their child's life. For them, financial support is only the beginning. They see themselves as a bulwark of safety for their child, providing a sense of security and stability by sheer virtue of "being there" in all the material, physical, and emotional senses that the term implies. Their children represent a source of love and belonging that many of them did not feel from their own fathers. They want to give their children a sense of emotional support and love that some of them did not have. The theme of fathers as builders of a stable and secure childhood is consistent with the concept of accessibility and responsibility articulated by Lamb et al. (1987) through the emphasis on physical and emotional presence. The clear intent to "be there" raises questions for researchers, practitioners, and policymakers about the best way to ensure their continuing presence beyond their children's early childhood. Here the Doherty (Doherty et al., 1998) framework may lend some insight in defining, measuring, and predicting those fathers who are most at risk of falling short of their own best intentions. Qualitative studies of low-income African American fathers provide strong evidence that employment and financial support are seen by mothers, the community, and fathers themselves as the "admission ticket" enabling them to be involved with their children (Jarrett, Roy, & Burton, 2002). Programs focusing on providing job training for fathers respond to this issue (Mincy & Pouncy, 2002). But for those fathers who remain in unstable economic circumstances, programs and policies that "unhook" access to their children from their ability to pay may enable some men to continue to "be there" for their children regardless of their economic circumstances.

Another clear message from these fathers is that teaching and molding their child is a central feature of their fatherhood role. For some, this meant emphasizing education and learning; for others, it meant imparting important values about "right and wrong" and how to get along with others in life. Within our theme of physical care and caregiving, the notion of "spending time" and taking their children on outings also had an underlying teaching intent. Fathers were also keenly aware of the teaching effect of their mere presence — the importance of their actions as role models for their children. For researchers, the theme of fathers as teachers is already a central part of the research agenda, especially with respect to fathers' contributions to child development as well as fathers' influence on successful educational experience. The emphasis by these fathers on teaching values such as work ethic and respect for others, and shaping personality traits such as self-reliance, suggests that studies of resilience in high-risk children might be informed by exploring the role of fathers and father figures in shaping the ability of young children to weather the challenges of poverty and violence in their lives. For practitioners, the recognition by these fathers of their teaching role is encouraging for the prospects of bringing these men into parent training and family development services. Explicitly linking the parent training curriculum into the kinds of teaching goals fathers espouse may make these programs more attractive to fathers. For more implications for practitioners, see an analysis of father involvement in EHS programs and fathers' responses to those initiatives reported by Raikes, Roggman, and Summers (2005). Given the strong value orientation of these fathers toward the types of characteristics and skills they hope to imbue in their children, EHS programs may also want to consider building linkages with other social institutions, including the religious community, to enhance the comfort of these fathers with their involvement in services for their child and family.

Some of these fathers had made the transition from more traditional father roles to the more modern role of coparent, meaning they shared every aspect of the parenting role with their child's mother (E. H. Pleck & Pleck, 1997). The emphasis by these men on providing love, emotional support, and a nurturing environment is one example. As another example, many of the fathers in this study talked of sharing fully the responsibilities of daily care of their children. For some of these low-income families, in fact, the parents were meeting their child care needs by working alternate shifts (one working days, the other evenings), meaning that some low-income fathers became primary caregivers for at least part of every working day. J. H. Pleck (1997) cited federal surveys of child care arrangements and concluded that as many as one fourth of fathers with children under age 5 provided primary child care for their children while the mothers were working. Research about the impacts of mothers' employment on father involvement suggested a complex picture; increases in accessibility and involvement in terms of sheer hours per day did not always result in greater direct engagement of fathers with their children (J. H. Pleck, 1997). The role of many fathers as direct caregivers, either while their partners are working or otherwise during substantial parts of the day, suggests a critical need for practitioners to reach these fathers and enhance their engagement with their children.

The men in our study displayed an obvious and strong attachment to their children. They believe it is their responsibility to provide a secure nest to foster their children's health and happiness. From the viewpoint of these interviews, taken at the time of their child's second birthday, these fathers are imbued with a strong sense of resolve to fulfill their commitments. But as researchers, practitioners, and policymakers, we know that not all these low-income fathers will be able keep those commitments as their child grows older and the family encounters more of the challenges associated with poverty. It is the task of social policymakers and service providers to develop constructive solutions to support these fathers to maintain their resolve.

AFFILIATIONS AND ADDRESSES

Jean Ann Summers, Beach Center on Disabilities, University of Kansas, 1200 Sunnyside, Room 3136, Lawrence, KS 66045. E-mail: jsummers@ku.edu. Kimberly Boller is at Mathematica Policy Research, Inc. Rachel F. Schiffman is at the University of Wisconsin–Milwaukee. Helen H. Raikes is at The Gallup Organization/University of Nebraska.

ACKNOWLEDGMENTS

The findings reported here are based on research conducted as part of the national Early Head Start Research and Evaluation Project funded by the Administration on Children, Youth and Families (ACYF), U.S. Department of Health and Human Services under contract 105–95–1936 to Mathematica Policy Research, Princeton, NJ, and Columbia University's Center for Children and Families, Teachers College, in conjunction with the Early Head Start Research Consortium. The Consortium consists of representatives from 17 programs participating in the evaluation, 15 local research teams, the evaluation contractors, and ACYF. Research institutions in the Consortium (and principal researchers) include Administration for Children and Families (Rachel Chazan-Cohen, Judith Jerald, Esther Kresh, Helen H. Raikes, and Louisa Tarullo); Catholic University of America (Michaela Farber, Lynn Milgram Mayer, Harriet Liebow, Christine Sabatino, Nancy Taylor, Elizabeth Timberlake, and Shavaun Wall); Columbia University (Lisa Berlin, Christy Brady-Smith, Jeanne Brooks-Gunn, and Alison Sidle Fuligni); Harvard University (Catherine Ayoub, Barbara Alexander Pan, and Catherine Snow); Iowa State University (Dee Draper, Gayle Luze, Susan McBride, and Carla Peterson); Mathematica Policy Research (Kimberly Boller, Ellen Eliason Kisker, John M. Love, Diane Paulsell, Christine Ross, Peter Schochet, Cheri Vogel, and Welmoet van Kammen); Medical University of South Carolina (Richard Faldowski, Gui-Young Hong, and Susan Pickrel); Michigan State University (Hiram

Fitzgerald, Tom Reischl, and Rachel Schiffman); New York University (Mark Spellmann and Catherine Tamis-LeMonda); University of Arkansas (Robert Bradley, Mark Swanson, and Leanne Whiteside-Mansell); University of California, Los Angeles (Carollee Howes and Claire Hamilton); University of Colorado Health Sciences Center (Robert Emde, Jon Korfmacher, JoAnn Robinson, Paul Spicer, and Norman Watt); University of Kansas (Jane Atwater, Judith Carta; and Jean Ann Summers); University of Missouri–Columbia (Mark Fine, Jean Ispa, and Kathy Thornburg); University of Pittsburgh (Beth Green, Carol McAllister, and Robert McCall); University of Washington School of Education (Eduardo Armijo and Joseph Stowitschek); and University of Washington School of Nursing (Kathryn Barnard and Susan Spieker), and Utah State University (Lisa Boyce and Lori Roggman). The authors thank the Consortium reviewers who commented on earlier drafts of this article under the guidelines of the Early Head Start Research Consortium publications polices. The authors express appreciation for the involvement of the children, families, staff, and Early Head Start program directors from the research sites for their dedication to the national study. The content of this publication does not necessarily reflect the views or policies of the Department of Health and Human Services, and mention of trade names, commercial products, or organizations does not imply endorsement by the U.S. Government.

REFERENCES

Allen, S. M., & Hawkins, A. J. (1999). Maternal gatekeeping: Mothers' beliefs and behaviors that inhibit greater father involvement in family work. *Journal of Marriage and the Family, 61*, 199–212.

Anfara, V. A., Brown, K. M., & Mangione, T. L. (2002). Qualitative analysis on stage: Making the research process more public. *Educational Researcher, 37*, 28–38.

Cabrera, N., Ryan, R., Shannon, J., Brookes-Gunn, J., Vogel, C., Raikes, H., et al. (2004). Low-income fathers' involvement in their toddlers' lives: Biological fathers from the Early Head Start National Research and Evaluation Study. *Fathering, 2*, 5–30.

Child Support Performance and Incentive Act of 1998, 42 U.S.C. § 651 et. seq.

Crouter, A. C., Bumpus, M. F., Head, M. R., & McHale, S. M. (2001). Implications of overwork and overload for the quality of men's family relationships. *Journal of Marriage and Family, 63*, 404–416.

Doherty, W. J., Kouneski, E., & Erickson, M. F. (1998). Responsible fathering: An overview and conceptual framework. *Journal of Marriage and the Family, 60*, 277–292.

Harold-Goldsmith, R., Radin, N., & Eccles, J. S. (1988). Objective and subjective reality: The effects of job loss and financial stress on fathering behaviors. *Family Perspective, 22*, 309–325.

Hawkins, A. J., & Dollahite, D. C. (1997). *Generative fathering: Beyond deficit perspectives*. Thousand Oaks, CA: Sage.

Jarrett, R. L., Roy, K. M., & Burton, L. M. (2002). Fathers in the "hood": Insights from qualitative research on low-income African–American men. In C. S. Tamis-LeMonda & N.

Cabrera (Eds.), *Handbook of father involvement: Multidisciplinary perspectives* (pp. 211–248). Mahwah, NJ: Lawrence Erlbaum Associates, Inc.

Jones, L. (1991). Unemployed fathers and their children: Implications for policy and practice. *Child and Adolescent Social Work Journal, 8*, 101–116.

Lamb, M. E., Pleck, J. H., Charnov, E. L., & Levine, J. A. (1987). A biosocial perspective on paternal behavior and involvement. In J. Lancaster, J. Altmann, A. Rossi, & L. Sherrod (Eds.), *Parenting across the lifespan: Biosocial dimensions* (pp. 111–142). New York: Aldine de Gruyter.

LaRossa, R., & Reitzes, D. (1993). Continuity and change in middle class fatherhood: 1925–1939: The culture-conduct connection. *Journal of Marriage and the Family, 55*, 455–468.

Marsiglio, W., Amato, P., Day, R., & Lamb, M. (2000). Scholarship on fatherhood in the 1990s and beyond. *Journal of Marriage and the Family, 62*, 1173–1191.

McBride, B. A., & Rane, T. R. (1998). Parenting alliance as a predictor of father involvement: An exploratory study. *Family Relations, 47*, 229–236.

McBride, B. A., Schoppe, S. J., & Rane, T. R. (2002). Child characteristics, parenting stress, and parental involvement: Fathers versus mothers. *Journal of Marriage and Family, 64*, 998–1011.

Miles, M. B., & Huberman, A. M. (1994). *Qualitative data analysis: An expanded sourcebook* (2nd ed.). Thousand Oaks, CA: Sage.

Mincy, R. B., & Pouncy, H. W. (2002). The responsible fatherhood field: Evolution and goals. In C. S. Tamis-LeMonda & N. Cabrera (Eds.), *Handbook of father involvement: Multidisciplinary perspectives* (pp. 555–597). Mahwah, NJ: Lawrence Erlbaum Associates, Inc.

Pleck, E. H., & Pleck, J. H. (1997). Fatherhood ideals in the United States: Historical dimensions. In M. E. Lamb (Ed.), *The role of the father in child development* (3rd ed., pp. 33–48). New York: Wiley.

Pleck, J. H. (1997). Paternal involvement: Levels, sources, and consequences. In M. E. Lamb (Ed.), *The role of the father in child development* (3rd ed., pp. 66–103). New York: Wiley.

Raikes, H. H., Roggman, L., & Summers, J. A. (2005). Father involvement in Early Head Start Programs. *Fathering: A Journal of Theory, Research, and Practice About Men as Fathers, 3*(1), 29–58.

Salem, D. A., Zimmerman, M. A., & Notaro, P. C. (1998). Effects of family structure, family process, and father involvement on psychosocial outcomes among African–American adolescents. *Family Relations, 47*, 331–341.

Summers, J. A., Raikes, H., Butler, J., Spicer, P., Pan, B., Shaw, S., et al. (1999). Low-income fathers' and mothers' perceptions of the father role: A qualitative study in four early Head Start communities. *Infant Mental Health Journal, 20*.

PARENTING: SCIENCE AND PRACTICE
April–September 2006 Volume 6 Numbers 2 & 3 Pages 167–188

Fathering in Infancy: Mutuality and Stability Between 8 and 16 Months

Jacqueline D. Shannon, Catherine S. Tamis-LeMonda, and Natasha J. Cabrera

SYNOPSIS

Objective. This longitudinal investigation explores how fathers engage with their infants, how their behaviors matter within and across developmental time, and how demographic and social factors affect the quality of the father – infant relationship. ***Design.*** Participants were 74 racially and ethnically diverse, low-income fathers from the Father and Newborn Study (FANS) and their 8- and 16-month-old infants (36 boys, 38 girls). Father – infant interactions were videotaped during semistructured free play in participants' homes. The quality of father – infant interactions was assessed using Likert-type ratings of fathers' and infants' behaviors. Fathers also rated their relationship with their infant's mother. ***Results.*** Two factors of father engagement emerged at each age (Responsive – Didactic and Negative – Overbearing), 2 factors of infant behavior at 8 months (Mastery, Social - Communicative), and 3 factors of infant behavior at 16 months (Mastery, Social, and Communicative). Responsive – Didactic fathering was concurrently associated with infant behaviors at both ages, although fathering at 8 months only marginally predicted infant 16-month Social behaviors. Fathers who were older, more educated, married to their partners, and who had higher incomes were more Responsive – Didactic at 8 months. Fathers' age and the quality of the mother – father relationship predicted fathers' Responsive – Didactic behaviors at the 16-month assessment. ***Conclusions.*** Fathers' responsiveness is important to infants' social and communicative behaviors, and the mother – father relationship influences fathering during the formative period of infancy.

INTRODUCTION

Infancy is a period of enormous parental investment (Bornstein & Tamis-LeMonda, 2001). Parents nurture, comfort, care for, and teach their infants virtually every day, and the quality of these parent – infant interactions exerts enduring influence on children's social and cognitive development. Daily activities between caregivers and their babies form the basis for infants' developing attachment, communication, and social cognition, as babies increasingly appreciate that experiences and intentions can be shared with trusted others. Although these developmental processes characterize mother – infant and father – infant relationships alike, the parenting literature continues to be dominated by research on mother – infant interactions in predominantly middle-income, two-parent families. This longitudinal study of low-income fathers and their infants addresses this gap by offering a descriptive account of the nature, consequences, and determinants of fathers' behaviors with their 8- and 16-month-old infants.

Fathering in Infancy

The focus on father – infant engagement is of theoretical and practical significance. From a theoretical standpoint, infancy is a period of rapid change; fathers and mothers alike must adjust their behaviors daily in response to infants' growing needs and competencies. Fathers who are able to sensitively accommodate infants' emerging abilities are thought to promote secure infant attachments and to further their own enjoyment of and commitment to their roles as fathers (Lamb & Lewis, 2004). Fathers' sensitivity and responsiveness toward their infants and young toddlers are associated with young children's social competencies and language and cognitive abilities, both concurrently and predictively (Black, Dubowitz, & Starr, 1999; Lamb & Lewis, 2004; Shannon, Tamis-LeMonda, London, & Cabrera, 2002; Tamis-LeMonda, Shannon, Cabrera, & Lamb, 2004).

From a practical standpoint, infancy is a time of unparalleled opportunity for practitioners and policymakers to support men who are invested in their "new" roles as fathers. Findings from the Fragile Families and Child Wellbeing study demonstrate that 80% of low-income unmarried fathers are present and express firm intentions to remain involved in their newborns' lives (Carlson & McLanahan, 2002). However, a measurable proportion of fathers who are initially committed and involved become disengaged later in infancy and the toddler years (Lerman, 1993; Perloff & Buckner, 1996). Therefore, researchers should aim to better understand fathering among those low-income men who are still present in their infants' lives before declines in father involvement begin. Preliminary research in our laboratory reveals that fathers' behaviors during pregnancy and birth (e.g., accompanying mother to prenatal visits, being present at the newborn's birth) predict their presence and involvement in their children's lives 3 years later (Shannon, Tamis-LeMonda, Cabrera, & Lamb, 2003). A first step toward promoting healthy father – infant relationships is to document how fathers engage with their infants, how their engagement matters within and across developmental time, and how demographic and social factors contribute to the quality of the father – infant relationship. The Father and Newborn Study (FANS) offers unprecedented data on the behaviors of present, positively involved, low-income fathers and their babies that enable us to begin tackling these complex questions.

Assessing Father – Infant Interactions

Our first goal was to describe father – infant interactions at 8 and 16 months and to explore associations between these father and infant behaviors. In these assessments, we contrasted didactic, responsive, and positive modes of fathering with behaviors that were overbearing and negative in affect. Didactic behaviors were those in which fathers encouraged infants to engage and understand the environment outside the dyad by focusing the infant's attention on properties, objects, or events in the immediate surroundings as well as introducing, mediating, and interpreting the external world, describing, and demonstrating, or providing opportunities to observe, imitate, learn, and the like (Bornstein, 2002). Responsive behaviors encompassed the contingent, prompt, and appropriate reactions that fathers displayed to infants' verbal and nonverbal initiatives. Positive behaviors were affective displays that were positive or comforting. Overbearing behaviors were those in which fathers interfered with or inhibited their infants' behaviors, and negative behaviors were those in which fathers displayed negative affect either facially or vocally. These contrasting forms of behavior have been the focus of mother – infant engagement for decades, and have formed the basis for widely used taxonomies of parenting (Bornstein, 1995; Bornstein & Tamis-LeMonda, 2001). Although these behaviors capture distinct aspects of parenting, they often relate to one another. For example, parents' responsiveness has been strongly associated with didactic and positive behaviors; therefore, these behaviors have frequently been combined. Similarly, parents' overbearing behaviors have related to negativity, thus, these behaviors have also been combined (e.g., Love et al., 2002; Tamis-LeMonda et al., 2004).

Research in our laboratory has demonstrated the beneficial effects of Responsive – Didactic fathering for 2- and 3-year-old children (Shannon et al., 2002; Tamis-LeMonda et al., 2004). However, no studies have explored the predictive validity of these modes of engagement in fathers during the infancy period. Infants might show differential reactions to specific parental behaviors in mothers versus fathers (e.g., infants may show more tolerance of intrusiveness in fathers than in mothers). There is also some evidence suggesting that infants might develop somewhat different patterns of engagement with their fathers, due to spending less time with them (Pleck,

1997) in different developmental contexts (e.g., play; Lamb, Frodi, Hwang, & Frodi, 1983; Roggman, Boyce, & Cook, 2002).

The coding of infant behaviors paralleled behaviors observed in fathers. Social behaviors were those that were directed toward interpersonal interactions — smiles, coos, and face-to-face interactions. Infants' responsiveness captured behaviors that were participatory and sensitive to their fathers' overtures. Infants' play and communicative behaviors paralleled didactic behaviors in fathers — vocalizations, verbalizations, gestures, and interest in and engagement with toys.

Determinants of Father Involvement

Our second goal was to examine particular determinants of father involvement within and across the 8- to 16-month period. Fathering is affected by multiple interacting systems, operating at different levels over the life course, including personal characteristics (e.g., motivation, skills, and self-confidence), children's characteristics (e.g., temperament, gender), social contextual factors (e.g., relationships with partners and extended family members, socioeconomic opportunity, cultural ideologies), and institutional practices and public policies (e.g., welfare support, child support enforcement; Belsky, 1984; Lamb & Tamis-LeMonda, 2004; Tamis-LeMonda & Cabrera, 2002). For purposes of this study, we focus on demographic characteristics of fathers (income, education, and age) as well as the mother – father relationship (father residency, marital status, and the quality of the mother – father relationship).

Characteristics of fathers. Fathers who are employed and educated are more likely to be involved with their children while they live with them as well as after divorce or nonmarital births, perhaps because they are better able to support their children economically (Rangarajan & Gleason, 1998; Stier & Tienda, 1993; Sullivan, 1993). Additionally, older fathers are more able to provide for their children than are younger fathers, given that older fathers are more likely to be educated and employed (Lerman, 1993). Older fathers are also more involved with their infants and children and are found to display greater sensitivity in their interactions than younger fathers (Fagan, 1996; Gavin et al., 2002).

Mother – father relationship. The roles that fathers play in family life often depend on mothers' attitudes, expectations, and the quality of the mother – father relationship (Allen & Hawkins, 1999). Mothers have been found to gatekeep nonresidential fathers' access to children, and mothers often constrain and define the roles and responsibilities of both residential and nonresidential fathers (Cabrera, Tamis-LeMonda, Bradley, Hofferth, & Lamb, 2000; Lamb & Tamis-LeMonda, 2004). In our own work, we found that fathers who reside with their partners and children are more involved with their children than their nonresidential counterparts because they have more access to their children on a daily basis (Cabrera et al, 2004). Residential fathers are also more likely to engage in sensitive behaviors than nonresidential fathers (Brophy-Herb, Gibbons, Omar, & Schiffman, 1999).

Positive paternal influences are also more likely to occur when fathers establish positive relationships with the mothers of their children. Warm and close mother – father relationships are linked to greater paternal involvement (McKenry, Price, Fine, & Serovich, 1992). In contrast, unmarried fathers in unstable or hostile relationships with their child's mother are more likely to be uninvolved (Edin & Lein, 1997; Gavin et al., 2002) and to display negative involvement with their children (Coley & Chase-Lansdale, 2000). A substantial literature shows that marital discord and conflict mediates the association between father engagement and child well-being (Cummings, Goeke-Morey, & Raymond, 2004).

This Study

This study uses data from FANS of the Early Head Start Research and Evaluation Project. FANS was designed to address the following questions: (1) How do different degrees, timing, and intensity of father involvement influence infant and toddler development? (2) How do fathers interact and become involved with their newborns? (3) How do fathers' relationships with their children's mothers relate to their children's development? and (4) How does early father involvement predict later parental involvement? This study examines the quality of father – infant engagement when infants were 8 and 16 months and fathers' behaviors were related to infants' behaviors within and across age. In addition, fathers' demographic characteristics and the quality of the mother – father relationship were examined in relation to fathers' engagement at both assessments and to patterns of fathering over time. We contrasted two models in our analysis (Bornstein, 1989a, 1989b, 1995; Bradley, Caldwell, & Rock, 1988). To test a "contemporary" model, we asked whether fathers' behaviors and infant behaviors at 8 and 16 months related concurrently. To test an "early effects" model, we asked whether the quality of father – infant engagement at 8 months uniquely predicted infant behaviors at 16 months after controlling for fathers' concurrent behaviors. Fathers and infants were observed during free play, in light of the prominence of play in father – infant interactions. Fathers spend greater proportions of time in play with their young infants than do mothers, and paternal playfulness and relative novelty is thought to enhance fathers' salience to their infants and young children (e.g., Lamb et al., 1983; Roggman et al., 2002).

METHODS

Participants

Unlike the other Early Head Start father substudies, not all the families in FANS were part of the Early Head Start evaluation; some were recruited to participate from other infant and toddler programs that also provided comprehensive services to families. As in the Father Involvement with Toddlers Substudy (FITS; described by Boller et al., this issue), mothers were recruited into the study first and were asked to help identify and contact fathers. Mothers were asked if they expected their child's biological father would rear their child with them. If the biological father was not involved in their child's life and not expected to rear their child, then mothers were asked if they were in a romantic relationship with a father figure for the child with whom they expected to rear their child. If a biological or a romantic father figure (usually the mother's boyfriend) was named, then researchers contacted the identified fathers by telephone and informed them of the research. A father visit was scheduled and written consent to participate in the study was obtained from fathers. Of the 265 families who completed a first interview, only 4% included men who were not the child's biological father.

Mother and father interviews were conducted when the children were 1, 3, 8, 16, and 24 months old. Fathers and children also participated in three brief videotaped interaction tasks when the children were 8, 16, and 24 months old. For the 8- and 16-month father visits, we intended to complete them when infants were 6 and 14 months old by initially contacting fathers when their infants were 4 and 12 months of age, however, actually scheduling visits took several months and infants, on average, were 8 and 16 months old when father interviews and videotaped interactions were completed. Many of the same questions asked of mothers were drawn from the parent interviews used in the Main Study of the Early Head Start Evaluation, and many of the questions asked of fathers were drawn from the FITS study. Additional questions included asking both mothers and fathers about the father's involvement during the pregnancy, the child's birth and the newborn period, and the quality of the mother – father relationship.

Of the initial 123 men participating in the videotaped portion of the FANS at 8 months, 74 fathers (60%) agreed to participate in the 16-month videotaped assessment. The final sample, therefore, comprised 74 fathers and their infants (36 boys and 38 girls).

Most father – infant dyads (78%) were from urban neighborhoods and came from diverse racial and ethnic backgrounds with the majority being Latin American (46%) or African American (36%). A smaller percentage of fathers were European American (15%) or Chinese American (3%). Sixty fathers spoke English, and 14 spoke another language (12 Spanish and 2 Cantonese). The majority of fathers (71%) had been living with their infants since birth, and they were unmarried (69%). About half (n = 39) were first-time fathers. At the time of the interview, fathers ranged from 16 to 39 years of age (M = 25, SD = 6.8). Their infants averaged 8.19 months (SD = 1.49) at the time of the 8-month assessment and 16.15 months (SD = 2.11) at the time of the 16-month assessment. Over a third, 36% (n = 27), of fathers completed 11 or fewer years of high school; 38% (n = 28) graduated from high school or received their government equivalency diploma; and 26% (n = 19) completed some college or graduated from college. All infants' mothers were low income and eligible to receive some form of governmental assistance (e.g., Medicaid, food stamps, WIC). Most of the fathers (8 months: 93%; 16 months: 85%) reported working full time or part time, and their mean monthly income was $1,251 ($SD$ = $970) at 8 months and $1,377 ($SD$ = $1040) at 16 months.

Overall, demographic characteristics of father – infant dyads who participated at both time points did not differ from those who only participated in the 8-month videotaped assessment. The exception was that Latin American fathers were more likely to participate at both time points than fathers from the other racial and ethnic groups, $\chi^2(2, N = 121) = 9.50, p < .01$.

Procedures

Father – infant videotaped interaction task. Dyads were videotaped during semistructured free play for 8 min at 8 months and 10 min at 16 and 24 months. They were provided with a standard set of age appropriate toys (8 months: a set of plastic rings, soft plastic book, musical ball, plastic colorful bolster with bells, and a brightly colored double-star fine motor toy; 16 and 24 months: three separate bags which included a book, a pizza set and telephone, and a farm with farm animals). Fathers were asked to sit on a mat with their children, to ignore the camera, and to do whatever was most natural to them. They were instructed to play only with the toys presented to them and to divide up the time as they chose.

Coding. The quality of father – infant interactions was assessed using the Caregiver – Child Affect, Responsiveness, and Engagement Scale (C-CARES;

Tamis-LeMonda, Rodriguez, Shannon, Ahuja, & Hannibal, 2002; Shannon et al., 2002), which rates various father, infant, and dyad behaviors on a 5-point Likert-type scale (1 = *behavior not observed* to 5 = *behavior constantly observed*). At 8 months, 18 father and 9 infant items were used, and at 16 months, 19 father and 13 infant items were used (see Table 1 for father items). Infant items were as follows: positive affect, negative affect, emotional regulation, participation with caregiver, responsiveness to caregiver, emotional attunement, persistence, toy play, and amount of communication. Additional infant items at 16 months were positive touch, negative touch, play sophistication, and quality of communication. These items were coded at 16 months and not at 8 months because of development in children's communication and play skills that occur around their first birthday.

Two trained coders reached 85% agreement (within 1 point) with 10 "gold standard tapes" before coding interactions separately. Ten percent of the remaining tapes were randomly assigned to one research assistant to ensure reliability. Interrater agreement ranged from 87% to 100% agreement (exact and within 1-point agreement). Correlational estimates of interrater reliability ranged from .71 to .97. Coders of father – infant engagement were fluent in the language of the participants. Coders were unaware of fathers' ratings of the quality of the mother – father relationship.

Demographics. Fathers were interviewed about their residency (0 = *nonresident*, 1 = *resident*), marital status (0 = *unmarried*, 1 = *married*), age, race and ethnicity, primary language, educational background, monthly income, and parity. Their infants' gender (0 = *boy*, 1 = *girl*) and age and their families' urban/rural residency (0 = *not urban*, 1 = *urban*) were gathered from mother interviews.

Mother – father relationship. The quality of fathers' relationship with their infants' mothers was based on two questions at 8 and 16 months. Fathers were asked to respond on a 5-point Likert-type scale (1 = *poor* to 5 = *excellent*) to the following question: "In general, how would you rate the quality of your relationship with (CHILD'S) mother?" They were asked to respond on a 4-point Likert-type scale to the following question: "In general, how supportive would you say that your infant's mother is of your being a father to (CHILD)?" (1 = *tries to prevent you from having a relationship with child* to 4 = *very supportive*). Fathers overwhelmingly viewed their relationship with their infants' mothers positively, as indicated by their high scores on each scale at two ages (i.e., Quality of relationship: 8 months, M = 3.80, SD = .52; 16 months, M = 3.85, SD = .43; and Supportiveness: 8 months, M = 4.03, SD = 1.02; 16 moths, M = 3.85, SD = 1.17). These four questions were converted to z-scores and combined into one scale that

TABLE 1
Father Behaviors

Behavior Items	Definitions	8 Months		16 Months	
		M	*SD*	*M*	*SD*
Positive affect	Display enjoyment, approval, or affection through facial expressions and tone of voice	3.62	1.13	3.50	1.06
Negative affect	Display disapproval, anger, or impatience through facial expressions and tone of voice	1.38	.77	1.31	.62
Positive touch	Amount and quality of gentle, playful touch using hands, face, or body	3.61	1.17	3.36	1.43
Negative touch	Amount and quality of forceful, abrupt touch using hands, face, or body	1.85	1.00	2.01	1.01
Positive verbal statements	Expression of approval, praise, and positive reinforcement	1.89	.91	2.62	1.42
Negative verbal statements	Expression of disapproval for noncompliance and negative behavior	1.50	.78	1.62	1.00
Teasing	Contradict infant's actions in a playful or antagonistic manner	1.84	1.06	1.53	.86
Participation with infant	Amount of involvement with the infant, not the quality	4.19	.95	4.42	.95
Responsiveness to nonverbal cues	Contingent and appropriate responsiveness to infant's nonverbal cues	3.27	1.13	2.68	1.20
Responsiveness to vocalizations	Contingent and appropriate responsiveness to infant's verbal cues	2.14	1.39	2.91	1.37
Emotional attunement	Emulate infant's emotions using voice, gestures, and facial expressions	2.50	1.21	1.92	1.06
Flexibility	Willingness to let the infant direct an activity	3.91	1.11	4.20	.89
Intrusiveness	Interrupt, restrict, or hover over the infant's play	2.39	1.19	2.15	.92
Structuring	Organize environment and materials to maximize infants' play and learning	3.73	1.08	3.73	1.25
Achievement orientation	Encourage cognitive achievement through directive teaching	2.22	1.14	2.07	1.08
Toy play	Amount of the father's play with the toys, not sophistication of play	3.54	1.09	3.77	.90
Play sophistication	Use of symbolic play as opposed to functional nonsymbolic play	—	—	1.74	.66
Amount of language	Amount of verbal stimulation provided, regardless of content and style	2.96	1.21	3.36	.99
Quality of language	Quality of verbal stimulation; level of explanatory verbal style	2.76	1.33	2.45	1.06

measured mother – father relationship quality, which demonstrated adequate internal consistency with a coefficient alpha of .73.

RESULTS

Descriptions of Father and Infant Behaviors

The means and standard deviations of 8- and 16-month father C-CARES items are presented in Table 1. At both ages, father and infant items displayed modest to strong variation.

Father behaviors. At both 8 and 16 months, fathers received the highest scores on positive items such as participation, flexibility, toy play, structuring, and positive affect. Their lowest scores were on the items of negative affect, negative verbal statements, and teasing. Patterns were similar across ages, although fathers received higher scores on positive verbal statements and language amount at the 16-month versus 8-month assessment, $ts(73) = -4.91$ and -3.18, $ps < .001$. Fathers received lower scores on teasing at 16 months and were more responsive to infants' vocalizations at 16 months; they were less responsive to infants' nonverbal cues and less emotionally attuned to their infants at the 16-month assessment, $ts(73) =$ 2.16, −3.45, 3.46, and 3.49, respectively, $ps < .05$. These mean level differences were likely explained by developmental changes in infants. Infants were beginning to communicate verbally by 16 months, and fathers met these changes with increased attentiveness to infants' vocalizations and less attentiveness to nonverbal forms of infant communication.

Infant behaviors. At both ages, infants received relatively high scores on toy play and persistence. They were rated lowest on negative affect and emotional attunement. The low scores on emotional attunement may be explained by the context of play; infants' attention to the toy materials might have inhibited emotional displays. Infants were more involved with and responsive toward their fathers, more emotionally regulated, persistent, involved in toy play, and communicative at 16 months, $ts(73)$, range −2.01 to −5.47, $ps < .05$.

Factor Analyses of Father and Infant Behavior

Exploratory factor analyses were conducted to examine whether the coded items might be reduced in a meaningful way. Consistent and interpretable solutions were identified for fathers and infants at both ages.

Father factor analyses. Two-factor solutions using principal component analysis with varimax rotation provided the most meaningful solutions for both 8-month and 16-month father behaviors on the C-CARES (see Table 2). These solutions paralleled those obtained in prior studies with other samples using the C-CARES when children were 8 months, 16 months, and 24 months of age (Shannon et al., 2002; Spellmann, Tamis-LeMonda, & Baumwell, 2000).

At both ages, the first factor, labeled Responsive – Didactic (12 items at 8 and 16 months), consisted of all positive items: positive affect, positive verbal statements, positive touch, participation, responsiveness to nonverbal cues, responsiveness to child vocalizations, emotional attunement, structuring, achievement orientation, toy play, amount of language, and quality of language and play sophistication (this item was only measured at 16

TABLE 2
Factor Analyses of Father Behaviors at 8 and 16 Months

	8-Month Factor Solution		16-Month Factor Solution	
Father Behavior Items	Responsive – Didactic	Negative – Overbearing	Responsive – Didactic	Negative – Overbearing
Positive affect	.76		.62	
Negative affect		.49		.64
Positive touch[a]	.32			
Negative touch		.62		.43
Positive verbal statements	.58		.46	
Negative verbal statements		.46		.42
Teasing		.62		.44
Participation with infant	.73		.53	
Responsiveness to nonverbal cues	.61		.69	
Responsiveness to vocalizations	.37		.21	
Emotional attunement	.56		.54	
Flexibility		–.86		–.85
Intrusiveness		.86		.75
Structuring	.52		.44	
Achievement orientation	.79		.39	
Toy play	.44		.55	
Play sophistication	—	—	.56	
Amount of language	.82		.72	
Quality of language	.77		.73	

Note: Extraction Method: Principal Component Analysis with Varimax Rotation.
[a]Positive touch only loaded on 8-month factor. Although the loading was low on the "Responsive – Didactic" factor (.32) at 8 months, we maintained this item because parental touch (e.g., holding) is a common parenting behavior during infancy.

months). The second factor, labeled Negative – Overbearing (6 items at 8 and 16 months), consisted of all negative behaviors: negative affect, negative verbal statements, negative touch, teasing, and intrusiveness, and negatively loaded on flexibility. A scree plot of the factor eigenvalues 3.8 and 1.9 supported the two-factor solution at 8 months and eigenvalues 4.0 and 2.5 supported the two-factor solution at 16 months. Two factors accounted for 45% of the item variance at 8 months and 34% of the item variance at 16 months.

The only inconsistencies in the factor loadings across the two ages were "positive touch" and "responsiveness to vocalizations." The "positive touch" item loaded on the Responsive – Didactic factor at 8 months. However, it did not load on either factor at 16 months and thus was eliminated from further analyses. The item "responsiveness to vocalizations" only weakly loaded on the Responsive – Didactic factor at 16 months. Nonetheless, we elected to retain this variable due to the predictive validity of responsiveness (Tamis-LeMonda, Bornstein, & Baumwell, 2001). The two scales at both ages demonstrated modest to good internal consistency with a coefficient alpha of .85 for Responsive – Didactic and .78 for Negative – Overbearing at 8 months, and .77 for Responsive – Didactic and .67 for Negative – Overbearing at 16 months.

At 8 months, fathers' scores on the Responsive – Didactic scale negatively related to their scores on the Negative – Overbearing scale, $r(74) = -.30, p < .01$. There was no association between fathers' scores on the two scales at 16 months, $r(74) = -.14$, *ns*. Fathers' scale scores were moderately stable over time, $r(74) = .44, p < .01$, for Responsive – Didactic; and $r(74) = .24, p < .05$, for Negative – Overbearing. Fathers' Responsive – Didactic scores did not vary at infant age of assessment; however, scores on Negative – Overbearing were negatively associated with infant age at 16 months, $r(74) = -.26, p < .05$.

Infant factor analyses. A two-factor solution using principal component analysis with varimax rotation for 8-month infant behaviors and a three-factor solution for 16-month behaviors on the C-CARES provided the most meaningful solutions. The two-factor solution at 8 months paralleled those identified in our prior studies of mother – infant interactions with their 8-month-olds (Spellmann et al., 2000). The three-factor solution at 16 months paralleled those identified in our prior research on father – child interactions with their 24-month-olds (Shannon et al., 2002).

The first factor at 8 and 16 months, labeled Mastery (four items at 8 months and five items at 16 months), consisted of emotional regulation, persistence, and involvement with toys, and negatively loaded on negative affect and negative touch (only measured at 16 months). The second factor at 8 months, labeled Social – Communication (five items), consisted of positive affect, participation with caregiver, responsiveness to caregiver, emotional attunement, and amount of communication. This second factor was split further into two factors at 16 months — Social and Communication. The Social factor (four items) consisted of positive affect, participation with caregiver, responsiveness to caregiver, and emotional attunement. The Communication factor (three items) consisted of amount of communication, quality of communication, and play sophistication. The item "positive touch," only at 16 months, did not load on any of the three factors and was excluded from further analyses.

A scree plot of the factor eigenvalues 3.8 and 1.9 supported the two-factor solution at 8 months and eigenvalues 3.9, 1.9, and 1.4 supported the three-factor solution at 16 months. The two factors at age 8 months accounted for 63% of the item variance at 8 months, whereas the three factors at 16 months accounted for 55% of the item variance. The scales at both ages demonstrated fair to strong internal consistency with coefficient alphas of .87 for Mastery and .76 for Social – Communication at 8 months; and .76 for Mastery, .64 for Social, and .64 for Communication at 16 months.

On average, infants frequently displayed mastery behaviors at both ages as indicated on their high Mastery scale scores (8 months: $M = 3.13$, $SD = .81$; 16 months: $M = 4.32$, $SD = .67$). Infants only rarely to occasionally displayed social and communicative behaviors at either age, as indicated by their low scores on the Social – Communication scale at 8 months ($M = 2.45$, $SD = .68$), and the Social ($M = 2.78$, $SD = .74$) and Communication ($M = 2.18$, $SD = .74$) scales at 16 months. Infant age at the 8-month assessment was unrelated to their scores on both child scale scores; however, age at the 16-month assessment was positively related to their mastery, cognitive, and social scale scores, $rs(74) = .34$ to $.42$, $p < .01$. Infant gender was unrelated to any scale score, $rs(74) = -.10$ to $.17$, *ns*.

Infants' Mastery and Social – Communication scale scores were positively associated, $r(74) = .38$, $p < .01$. At 16 months, toddler scores on Mastery, Social, and Communication scales all covaried, $rs(74) = .31$ to $.40$, $ps < .05$ and $.01$. Over time, infants' scale scores were unstable. Neither scale score at 8 months predicted any of the three infant scale scores at 16 months, $rs(74) = -.06$ to $.19$, *ns*.

Concurrent Associations Between Father and Infant Scales at 8 and 16 Months

Because infant age was related to all 16-month infant scale scores and to fathers' Negative – Overbearing scores, partial correlations between the father and infant scales were examined with infant age at assessment serving as a covariate. Fathers' scores on the Responsive – Didactic scale at 8 months related positively to infants' scores on the Social – Communication scale, $r(74) = .41$, $p < .01$. Fathers' scores on the Negative – Overbearing scale related negatively to infants' scores on the Social – Communication scale, $r(74) = -.21$, $p < .05$. Neither father scale related to infants' scores on the Mastery scale, $rs(74) = -.06$ and $-.05$, *ns*.

Similar associations between father and infant scales were obtained at 16 months. Fathers' scores on the Responsive – Didactic scale positively related to infants' scores on Social and Communication scales, $rs(74) = .55$ and .27, $ps < .05$ and .01. Fathers' Negative – Overbearing scale scores were unrelated to any of the three infant scales, $rs(74) = -.11$ to $-.06$, *ns*.

Predictive Associations from 8 to 16 Months

Father and infant scale scores at 8 months were examined in relation to father and infant scale scores at 16 months after covarying infant age. Fathers' scores on the 8-month Responsive – Didactic scale marginally predicted infant Social scale scores, $r\ (74) = .22$, $p = .07$. Fathers' scores on the Negative – Overbearing scale at the 8-month assessment did not predict any infant scale scores at 16 months, $rs\ (74) = -.12$ to .17, *ns*. Similarly, infant scale scores at 8 months did not predict father scale scores at 16 months, $rs(74) = -.07$ to .11, *ns*.

Determinants of Fathering

Fathers' age, education, income, residency, marital status, and quality of their relationship with the child's mother were next examined in relation to fathers' scale scores and to patterns of fathering over time. Infant age was covaried in these analyses because infant age related to fathers' scores on the Negative – Overbearing scale.

Bivariate correlations. At 8 months, older fathers and those married to their infants' mother received higher Responsive – Didactic scores and lower Negative – Overbearing scores, $rs(74) = -.21$ to .32, $ps < .05$. Fathers who resided with their infants received lower scores on the Negative – Overbearing scale, and fathers with more education and higher incomes received higher scores on the Responsive – Didactic Scale, $rs(74) = -.32$ to .28, $ps < .05$. At 16 months, fathers' age was marginally associated with their scores on the Responsive – Didactic scale, $r(74) = .22$, $p = .06$. The quality of the mother – father relationship was associated with fathers' scores on the Responsive – Didactic scale at 16 months, $r(74) = .26$, $p < .05$.

Multiple regressions. A series of regressions was conducted to examine predictors of father engagement at each age separately. At 8 months, infant age and 8-month Social – Communication behaviors, fathers' age, and the quality of the mother – father relationship were entered as predictors of fathers' Responsive – Didactic and Negative – Overbearing behaviors. We initially included all significant parent demographic characteristics (father age, education, income, and marital status for the 8 month Responsive – Didactic scale; father age, resident status, and marital status for 8 month Negative – Overbearing scale), but only father age was significant when other demographic characteristics were included in the same equation. Therefore, all other demographic variables were dropped from the equations after we controlled for father age.

Given that the vast majority of families in this study (97%) were in Early Head Start or another early intervention program, we did not include treatment status in our multivariate analyses. At 16 months, infant age, infants' 16-month behaviors, fathers' age, fathers' 8-month behaviors, and the quality of the mother – father relationship were entered as predictors (see Tables 3 and 4).

Significant results were obtained for all four models, particularly in relation to fathers' Responsive – Didactic behaviors. Specifically, fathers with older infants were less Responsive – Didactic at 8 months and less Negative – Overbearing at 16 months. Infants with higher scale scores had fathers who were more Responsive – Didactic and less Negative – Overbearing at both ages. After accounting for infant contributions, older fathers were more Responsive – Didactic and less Negative – Overbearing at 8 months, and fathers' earlier behaviors predicted their later behaviors.

TABLE 3
Prediction of Fathering at 8 Months

		8-Month Father Scales			
		Responsive – Didactic		Negative – Overbearing	
Step	Variables	β	ΔR^2	β	ΔR^2
1	Infant age	–.21*	.01	.02	.00
2	Significant Infant Scale		.16***		.06*
	Social – Communication	.44***		–.23	
3	Father age	.28**	.09**	–.21	.04
4	Mother - Father Relationship Quality	.15	.02	.04	.00
	R^2 total		.29		.10

Note: Beta weights presented are from the final regression equation.
$^{*}p \le .05$. $^{**}p \le .01$. $^{***}p \le .001$.

TABLE 4
Prediction of Fathering at 16 Months

		16-Month Father Scales			
		Responsive – Didactic		Negative – Overbearing	
Step	Variables	β	ΔR^2	β	ΔR^2
1	Infant age	–.05	.04	–.26*	.07*
2	Significant infant scales (block)		.29**		.00
	Social	.40**		.05	
	Communication	.21*		–.03	
3	Father age	.10	.04*	–.08	.02
4	Father scales (block)		.11**		.05*
	8 month Responsive – Didactic	.35**		—	—
	8 month Negative – Overbearing	—	—	.24*	
5	Mother - Father Relationship Quality	.21*	.04*	–.01	.00
	R^2 total		.52		.14

Note: Beta weights presented are from the final regression equation.
* $p \leq .05$. ** $p \leq .001$.

Finally, fathers who reported being in a higher quality relationship with their infants' mothers received higher Responsive – Didactic scores at 16 months, after controlling for all other predictors. At 8 months, the predictors explained 29% of the variance in fathers' Responsive – Didactic behaviors and 10% of the variance in fathers' Negative – Overbearing behaviors. By 16 months, the predictors explained 52% of the variance in fathers' Responsive – Didactic behaviors and 14% of fathers' Negative – Overbearing behaviors.

DISCUSSION

This longitudinal study builds on the growing body of research on low-income fathers by describing the nature and patterns of father – infant interactions when infants were 8 and 16 months. We examined associations between fathering and infant behaviors within and across time and explored demographics and the quality of the mother – father relationship as determinants of fathering.

This group of involved fathers interacted in ways that go beyond portrayals of fathers as "rough and tumble" playmates (see also Shannon et al., 2002). In the context of substantial individual variation, fathers were generally positive in their engagement with their infants at both ages, as indicated by their relatively high scores on participation, responsiveness, and flexibility, and relatively low scores on intrusiveness, negative affect, and negative touch.

Two meaningful factors of fathering were identified: Responsive – Didactic and Negative – Overbearing. This taxonomy of fathering mirrors extant findings on parenting styles in fathers and mothers (e.g., Baumwell, Tamis-LeMonda, & Bornstein, 1997; Black et al., 1999; Brophy-Herb et al., 1999; Heermann, Jones, & Witkoff, 1994). In infants, two meaningful factors were identified at 8 months, Mastery and Social – Communication, and three factors emerged at 16 months, Mastery, and the Social – Communication factor at 8 months split into two distinct factors: Social and Communication.

Within each of the two infant ages, fathers with higher scores on the Responsive – Didactic scale had infants who were more social and communicative in their engagement, supporting a contemporaneous model of influence. Fathers' scores on the Negative – Overbearing scale were either unrelated or inversely related to infants' engagement. The separate loading of variables onto Social versus Communicative factors at 16 but not at 8 months reflects the developmental transition that infants make in their verbal and play abilities between the two ages, although it is safe to say that associations likely reflect a bidirectional process. Fathers who display higher levels of responsive and didactic behaviors are likely to promote communication and social skills in their infants, and infants who display higher levels of communicative and social abilities promote sensitive, didactic interactions in their fathers, which may then influence infants' further developmental progress.

In this regard, it is surprising that fathers' Responsive – Didactic behaviors at 8 months only marginally predicted infants' 16-month behaviors, refuting an early effects model. The relative lack of associations between early father – infant engagement and later infant behaviors might reflect qualitative changes that occur in infants' capacities over this time frame, as well as the fact that fathering was only modestly stable across the 8-month period. Indeed, exploratory analyses (not presented in the report) shed light on this modest stability and offered an alternative interpretation to the lack of lagged father – infant associations. When the Responsive – Didactic and Negative – Overbearing scores of individual fathers were examined at the two ages, 51 of the 74 fathers (69%) displayed relatively continuous levels of fathering over time (i.e., 28 fathers received consistently high ratings on their fathering, and 23 received consistently low ratings on their fathering). However, the remaining 23 fathers fluctuated in the quality of their engagement over time, with 10 improving and 13 declining. Fathers who received consistently high scores and those who improved over time had infants who were more communicative and social at 16 months, supporting a contemporary model of fathering effects. These same parenting patterns were found in mothers of term and preterm infants (Landry, Smith, Swank, Assel, & Vellet, 2001). An optimistic interpretation of these data is that fathers' engagement in the second year can compensate for less than optimal engagement in the earlier infancy period when their fathers become or remain positively involved. Similarly, Landry and colleagues (2001) found that inconsistent or later maternal responsiveness is better for children than absence of responsiveness.

Our second goal was to examine whether fathers' demographics or the quality of the mother – father relationship predicted fathering within and across time. Fathers who were older, more educated, married to their partners, and who had higher incomes were better able to establish early connections with their infants, as reflected in positive associations between these variables and fathers' scores on the Responsive – Didactic scale at 8 months. By 16 months, however, fathers' age was the best single demographic predictor of fathering behavior.

Notably, the quality of the mother – father relationship positively predicted fathers' 16-month Responsive – Didactic behaviors over and above infant contributions, father age, and past Responsive – Didactic behaviors. Furthermore, the father – mother relationship reliably predicted patterns of fathers' engagement over time. Fathers who rated the quality of their relationships as high and who felt supported by their infant's mother were more likely to be either consistently high in their parenting quality or to increase in quality between the two ages. These findings parallel those on men from middle-income backgrounds, showing that those who feel supported by their partners in their role as father are more sensitive (Belsky, Youngblade, Rovine, & Volling, 1991; Brody, Pillegrini, & Sigel, 1986; Volling & Belsky, 1991) and playful (Levy-Shiff & Israelashvili, 1988) with their children than are fathers who are involved in less satisfying relationships. Similar results have been documented in low-income, adolescent parents (Lamb & Elster, 1985) and lower- to middle-income African American fathers (Ahmeduzzaman & Roopnarine, 1992). However, these associations between father – mother and father – infant relationships might be explained by variables not assessed in this study. For example, fathers in more supportive relationships with their partners were more responsive to their infants at 16 months, but not at 8 months. It may be that mother – father relationship quality predicts fathering over time, or alternatively, that fathers who are able to maintain "positive" relationships with their partners are those who are also able to remain "committed" (as in responsiveness) toward their infants a year after their babies' births. It may be that this ability to "commit" to relationships explains the covariance between the father – mother relationship and the father – infant relationship.

This study has several limitations that should be acknowledged. Participants were a select sample of men who were nominated for study inclusion by their partners and were themselves willing to participate. Consequently, assessments of fathering were likely biased toward positive engagement in this group of men. Moreover, these findings are limited to the settings and questions that were asked. For example, although the examination of fathering in the context of free play is important (Roggman et al., 2002), father – infant interactions in other settings might offer a different perspective on what fathers do with their infants. Similarly, evaluation of the mother – father relationship was based on two global questions that limit their scope and explanatory value, particularly in light of the modest sample size of 74 dyads. Nonetheless, these findings offer a glimpse into how involved, low-income fathers engage with and affect their infants' development over the foundational first to second year, and shed new light on the contributions that fathers' education, age, income, and support from partners make to early father – infant relationships.

AFFILIATIONS AND ADDRESSES

Jacqueline D. Shannon, Department of Applied Psychology, New York University, 239 Greene Street, Room 401F, New York, NY 10003. E-mail: jds225@nyu.edu. Catherine S. Tamis LeMonda is also at New York University. Natasha J. Cabrera is at the University of Maryland.

ACKNOWLEDGMENTS

We acknowledge our colleagues in the Early Head Start Father Studies Work Group, who are our partners in the commitment to better understand the roles of fathers in young children's lives. The Early Head Start Father Studies Work Group members represent the national Early Head Start evaluation contractor (Mathematica Policy Research and Columbia University), the funding agencies (the Ford Foundation; the Administration on Children, Youth and Families; and the National Institute of Child Health and Human Development, Office of the Assistant Secretary for Planning and Evaluation in Department of Health and Human Services), the local research universities participating in the Early Head Start Research Consortium, and program directors from the Early Head Start programs participating in the national evaluation. Catherine S. Tamis-LeMonda acknowledges funding from National Science Foundation for

New York University's Center for Research on Culture, Development and Education.

REFERENCES

Ahmeduzzaman, M., & Roopnarine, J. (1992). Sociodemographic factors, functioning styles, social support and fathers' involvement with preschoolers in African–American families. *Journal of Marriage and the Family, 54,* 699–701.

Allen, S. M., & Hawkins, A. J. (1999). Maternal gatekeeping: Mothers' beliefs and behaviors that inhibit greater father involvement in family work. *Journal of Marriage and Family, 61,* 199–212.

Baumwell, L., Tamis-LeMonda, C. S., & Bornstein, M. H. (1997). Maternal verbal sensitivity and child language comprehension. *Infant Behavior and Development, 20,* 247–258.

Belsky, J. (1984). The determinants of parenting: A process model. *Child Development, 55,* 83–96.

Belsky, J., Youngblade, L., Rovine, M., & Volling, B. (1991). Patterns of marital change and parent–child interaction. *Journal of Marriage and the Family, 53,* 487–498.

Black, M. M., Dubowitz, H., & Starr, R. H. (1999). African American fathers in low income, urban families: Development, behavior, and home environment of their three-year-olds. *Child Development, 70,* 967–978.

Bornstein, M. H. (1989a). Between caretakers and their young: Two modes of interaction and their consequences for cognitive growth. In M. H. Bornstein & J. S. Bruner (Eds.), *Interaction in human development* (pp. 197–214). Hillsdale, NJ: Lawrence Erlbaum Associates, Inc.

Bornstein, M. H. (Ed.). (1989b). *Maternal responsiveness: Characteristics and consequences.* San Francisco: Jossey-Bass.

Bornstein, M. H. (1995). Parenting infants. In M. H. Bornstein (Ed.), *Handbook of parenting, Vol. 1: Children and parenting* (2nd ed., pp. 3–39). Mahwah, NJ: Lawrence Erlbaum Associates, Inc.

Bornstein, M. H. (Ed.). (2002). *Handbook of parenting.* Mahwah, NJ: Lawrence Erlbaum Associates, Inc.

Bornstein, M. H., & Tamis-LeMonda, C. S. (2001). Mother–infant interaction. In G. Bremmer & A. Fogel (Eds.), *Blackwell handbook of infant development* (pp. 269–295). London: Blackwell.

Bradley, R. H., Caldwell, B. M., & Rock, S. L. (1988). Home environment and school performance: A ten-year follow-up and examination of three models of environmental action. *Child Development, 59,* 852–867.

Brody, G. H., Pillegrini, A. D., & Sigel, I. E. (1986). Marital quality and mother–child and father–child interactions with school-aged children. *Developmental Psychology, 22,* 291–296.

Brophy-Herb, H. E., Gibbons, C., Omar, M. A., & Schiffman, R. F. (1999). Low-income fathers and their infants: Interactions during teaching episodes. *Infant Mental Health Journal, 20,* 305–321.

Cabrera, N. J., Ryan, R., Shannon, J. D., Brooks-Gunn, J., Vogel, C., Raikes, H., et al., (2004). Fathers in the early head start national research and evaluation study: How are they involved with their children? *Fathering: A Journal of Theory, Research, and Practice About Men as Fathers, 2,* 5–30.

Cabrera, N. J., Tamis-LeMonda, C. S., Bradley, R. H., Hofferth, S., & Lamb, M. E. (2000). Fatherhood in the twenty-first century. *Child Development, 71,* 127–136.

Carlson, M., & McLanahan, S. (2002). Fragile families, father involvement and public policy. In C. S. Tamis-LeMonda & N. Cabrera (Eds.), *Handbook of father involvement:*

Multidisciplinary perspectives (pp. 555–597). Mahwah, NJ: Lawrence Erlbaum Associates, Inc.
Coley, R., & Chase-Lansdale, P. L. (2000). Father's involvement with their children over time. *Poverty Research News, 4,* 12–14.
Cummings, M. E., Goeke-Morey, M. C., & Raymond, J. (2004). Fathers in family context: Effects of marital quality and marital conflict. In M. E. Lamb (Ed.), *The role of the father in child development* (4th ed., pp. 196–221). Hoboken, NJ: Wiley.
Edin, K., & Lein, L. (1997). *Making ends meet: How single mothers survive welfare and low-wage work.* New York: Russell Sage Foundation.
Fagan, J. (1996). A preliminary study of low-income African American fathers' play interactions with preschool-age children. *Journal of Black Psychology, 22,* 7–19.
Gavin, L. E., Black, M. M., Minor, S., Abel, Y., Papas, M. A., & Bentley, M. A. (2002). Young, disadvantaged fathers' involvement with their infants: An ecological perspective. *Society for Adolescent Medicine, 31,* 266–276.
Heermann, J., Jones, L. C., & Witkoff, R. L. (1994). Measurement of parent behavior during interactions with their infants. *Infant Behavior and Development, 17,* 311–321.
Lamb, M. E., & Elster, A. B. (1985). Adolescent mother–infant–father relationships. *Developmental Psychology, 20,* 504–514.
Lamb, M. E., Frodi, M., Hwang, C. P., & Frodi, A. M. (1983). Effects of paternal involvement on infant preferences for mothers and fathers. *Child Development, 54,* 450–452.
Lamb, M. E., & Lewis, C. (2004). The development and significance of father–child relationships in two-parent families. In M. E. Lamb (Ed.), *The role of the father in child development* (4th ed., pp. 272–306). Hoboken, NJ: Wiley.
Lamb, M. E., & Tamis-LeMonda, C. S. (2004). The role of the father: An introduction. In M. E. Lamb (Ed.), *The role of the father in child development* (4th ed., pp. 1–31). Hoboken, NJ: Wiley.
Landry, S. H., Smith, K. E., Swank, P. R., Assel, M. A., & Vellet, S. (2001). Does early responsive parenting have a special importance for children's development or is consistency across early childhood necessary? *Developmental Psychology, 37,* 387–403.
Lerman, R. (1993). A national profile. In R. Lerman & T. Ooms (Eds.), *Young unwed fathers: Changing roles and emerging policies* (pp. 27–51). Philadelphia: Temple University Press.
Levy-Shiff, R., & Israelashvili, R. (1988). Antecedents of fathering: Some further exploration. *Developmental Psychology, 24,* 434–440.
Love, J. M., Kisker, E. E, Ross, C. M., Schochet, P. Z., Brooks-Gunn, J., Paulsell, D., et al., (2002). *Making a difference in the lives of infants and toddlers and their families: The impacts of Early Head Start. Executive summary* (Document No. PR02–30e). Princeton, NJ: Mathematica Policy Research.
McKenry, P. C., Price, S. J., Fine, M. A., & Serovich, J. (1992). Predictors of single, non-custodial fathers' physical involvement with their children. *Journal of Genetic Psychology, 153,* 305–320.
Perloff, J., & Buckner, J. (1996). Fathers of children of welfare: Their impact on child well-being. *American Journal of Orthopsychiatry, 66,* 557–571.
Pleck, J. H. (1997). Paternal involvement: Levels, origins, and consequences. In M. E. Lamb (Ed.), *The role of the father in child development* (3rd ed., pp. 66–103). New York: Wiley.
Rangarajan, A., & Gleason, P. (1998). Young unwed fathers of AFDC children: Do they provide support? *Demography, 35,* 175–186.
Roggman, L., Boyce, L., & Cook, J. (2002). Widening the lens: Viewing fathers in their infants' lives. In H. E. Fitzgerald, K. Karraker, & T. Luster (Eds.), *Infant development* (pp. 193–220). New York: Routledge Falmer.
Shannon, J. D., Tamis-LeMonda, C. S., Cabrera, N. J., & Lamb, M. E. (2003, April). *Determinants of father involvement: Presence/Absence and quality of engagement.* Paper presented at

the meeting of the Society of Research and Child Development Conference, Tampa Bay, FL.

Shannon, J. D., Tamis-LeMonda, C. S., London, K., & Cabrera, N. (2002). Beyond rough and tumble: Low-income fathers' interactions and children's cognitive development at 24 months. *Parenting: Science and Practice, 2,* 77–104.

Spellmann, M., Tamis-LeMonda, C. S., & Baumwell, L. (2000, June). *Mother–child relationships: Findings from the dyadic rating when children were six and fourteen months old.* Poster session presented at Head Start's Fifth National Research Conference, Washington, DC.

Stier, H., & Tienda, M. (1993). Are men marginal to the family? Insights from Chicago's inner city. In J. C. Hood (Ed.), *Men, work, and family* (pp. 23–44). Newbury Park, CA: Sage.

Sullivan, M. L. (1993). Young fathers and parenting in two inner-city neighborhoods. In R. I. Lerman & T. J. Ooms (Eds.), *Young unwed fathers: Changing roles and emerging policies* (pp. 52–73). Philadelphia: Temple University Press.

Tamis-LeMonda, C. S., Bornstein, M. H., & Baumwell, L. (2001). Maternal responsiveness and children's achievement of language milestones. *Child Development, 72,* 748–767.

Tamis-LeMonda, C. S., & Cabrera, N. (Eds.). (2002). *Handbook of father involvement: Multidisciplinary perspectives.* Mahwah, NJ: Lawrence Erlbaum Associates, Inc.

Tamis-LeMonda, C. S., Rodriguez, V., Shannon, J. D., Ahuja, P., & Hannibal, B. (2002). *Caregiver–Child affect, responsiveness, and engagement scale (C-CARES).* Unpublished manuscript.

Tamis-LeMonda, C. S., Shannon, J. D., Cabrera, N., & Lamb, M. E. (2004). Fathers and mothers at play with their 2- and 3-year olds: Contributions to language and cognitive development. *Child Development, 75,* 1806–1820.

Volling, B. L., & Belsky, J. (1991). Multiple determinants of father involvement during infancy in dual-earner and single-earner families. *Journal of Marriage and Family, 53,* 461–474.

PARENTING: SCIENCE AND PRACTICE Copyright © 2006, Lawrence Erlbaum Associates, Inc.
April–September 2006 Volume 6 Numbers 2 & 3 Pages 189–209

Relation Between Father Connectedness and Child Outcomes

Cheri A. Vogel, Robert H. Bradley, Helen H. Raikes, Kimberly Boller, and Jeffrey K. Shears

SYNOPSIS

Objective. We examine the relation between low-income fathers' presence in their children's lives and their children's early developmental outcomes using data from Early Head Start. ***Design.*** We grouped 1,930 children into 5 "classes" using maternal reports of fathers' presence and connectedness with the child. We developed the 5 mutually exclusive classes based on biological relatedness, residence in the home or frequency of contact, and stability of the relationship over time. We regressed 6 child outcomes on these classes of father connectedness (controlling for covariates). We also examined differences by race and ethnicity and ran the same regression models within the 3 major racial and ethnic groups. ***Results.*** Children with resident or involved nonresident biological fathers showed higher levels of self-regulation and lower levels of aggression than children with unstable father connections. Relations seemed most straightforward for European Americans and somewhat for Latin Americans, among whom a consistent biological father presence was associated with positive child developmental outcomes. Children with involved nonresident biological fathers were better off than children who had transient relationships with their fathers. These relations did not hold as consistently for African Americans. ***Conclusions.*** On average, frequent contact with a biological father is beneficial to children's development; however, relations appear to differ by race and ethnicity. Models that are valid and predictive for families from all racial and ethnic groups are needed, and programs developed that address individual needs and enhance development of all children.

INTRODUCTION

The significance of fathers and fathering for children's well-being has long been a focus of research. Interest in the role of the fathers has intensified in the wake of demographic and cultural shifts that have resulted in large numbers of single-parent (primarily female-headed) households. Many researchers have found the absence of a father to be associated with an array of child problems, including poor adjustment, behavioral difficulties, poor school achievement, and poor peer relationships (Amato, 1993; Amato & Keith, 1991; Biller, 1982; Blankenhorn, 1995; Hines, 1997). In response to information about the potential importance of fathers, myriad public policy initiatives have been advanced to understand, encourage, and facilitate fathers' involvement with their children, in programs that serve children and their families, and in marriage (Curran & Abrams, 2000).

Despite notable efforts to study fathering, much remains to be learned about the influence of fathers on children's development. Some research suggests that fathers make a unique contribution to children's well-being above and beyond what mothers contribute (England & Folbre, 2002; Graham & Beller, 2000; Lamb, 2002; Palkovitz, 2002). However, much of that research involved intact, European American, middle-class families and small samples of convenience. Knowledge about poor non-European American fathers is very limited, a situation that creates problems because public policy initiatives are aimed at encouraging father involvement in low-income families. This article attempts to answer some questions about relations between low-income fathers' presence in their children's lives and their children's early developmental outcomes using the large sample and unique data available from the Early Head Start study.

In this study, we depart from traditional classifications of father presence and relatedness to children in that low-income men (particularly those of minority status) who play a fathering role to children tend to vary greatly with respect to their relationship with the child (Cabrera, Tamis-LeMonda, Bradley, Hofferth, & Lamb, 2000). Accordingly, we adopt a broader perspective, focusing on the degree of father connectedness to the child. This perspective is multidimensional, one that simultaneously considers biological relatedness, residential status, amount of time spent with the child, and temporal stability of the relationship. Jointly, these factors determine the father's degree of connectedness to the child, and it is this degree of connectedness that is presumed to determine how much the father is likely to influence child well-being. Our research objectives were (1) to classify fathers according to their degree of connectedness with their child, and (2) to examine relations between these levels of connectedness and children's developmental outcomes.

We would expect that children in stable, intact, biological families, with presumably the most contact with their fathers, would have the best outcomes (e.g., Pollack & Ginther, 2003). Although we expect that children whose contact with their biological father is less stable or whose contact is mostly with a social father (father figure) would fare less well than children in intact biological families, it is less clear whether contact, even if sporadic, with a biological father would be more or less beneficial than similar contact with a father figure. However, we place biological relatedness ahead of residential status in terms of likely association. We hypothesize this because partnerships that develop soon after birth between mothers and men who are not biologically related to a child may signify less stable relationships of uncertain duration. Furthermore, research on step families shows that children living with a biological parent and a step parent fare no better than children in single parent families, and worse than children living with two biological parents (Pollack & Ginther, 2003).

In addition to our overarching questions about the general relations between classes of father connectedness and child outcomes, we considered it useful to examine relations between our classes of connectedness and child outcomes within racial and ethnic groups. This interest stemmed from observations that fatherhood and family relationships may have different meanings for different groups, which, in turn, may affect relations between father connectedness and child outcomes. Ethnographic accounts of male parenting in regard to a man's biological relatedness to a child, and a man's legal relatedness to the child's mother, suggest variations in the paternal role across racial and ethnic groups in the United States (Hofferth, 1984). In previous analyses of developmental measures from the Early Head Start National Evaluation Study, racial and ethnic differences were observed in child measures (Administration for Children and Families, 2002). In early exploratory work for this article, we also noted marked differences across racial and ethnic groups on characteristics such as mothers' education, receipt of welfare, and incidence of marriage, among others (see Table 1).

Our objective was to develop a scheme for quantifying and defining classes of father connectedness to the lives of their children and to apply it to our sample. As noted in the introductory article in this Special Issue, the Early Head Start evaluation yielded rich data with information on many aspects of family life, parenting behavior, and child development, and it includes information provided by mothers about the fathers and father figures in their children's lives in a large sample of low-income families (Boller et al., this issue). In contrast to other articles in this Special Issue that used father reports from the Father Involvement with Toddlers Study (FITS), we used data from the main study (maternal reports about fathers) to inform our models for three reasons: (1) they constituted the largest possible sample, (2) they contained information collected at up to three time points, and (3) they included families with absent fathers, a group of interest. As part of the standard interview that occurred when children were 14, 24, and 36 months old, mothers were asked about the men who played a fathering role in the lives of focus children. The process for fathers to be interviewed or videotaped was complex. First, mothers had to be interviewed, then interviewed mothers had to identify the father or father figure and to

TABLE 1
Sample Characteristics Overall and Within Race and Ethnicity

Characteristic								
	Percentage							
		Overall		European American		African American		Latin American
Classes of father connectedness								
Stable resident biological father		39		46		16		56
Nonresident biological father		22		17		33		13
Stable father figure presence		5		7		4		4
Unstable father presence[a]		31		26		42		23
No father presence		4		3		4		4
Background characteristics (Control variables)								
Early Head Start program		53		52		52		55
Race								
European American[a]		39		—		—		—
African American		33		—		—		—
Latin American		23		—		—		—
Mother's education (years)								
Less than 12[a]		45		30		45		71
12 or GED		29		37		31		16
More than 12		26		33		24		13
Teen mother		37		30		50		32
Urban residence		56		39		65		68
Family received welfare		51		50		64		38
Boy		51		49		51		55
	M	*SD*	*M*	*SD*	*M*	*SD*	*M*	*SD*
Parent – child dysfunctional interaction	17.76	6.27	17.64	5.50	17.68	6.72	18.30	7.07
Parenting distress	25.16	9.62	24.61	9.13	25.47	10.05	25.74	9.99
N	1841 – 1930		718 – 744		603 – 624		410 – 443	

[a]Represents the omitted or reference category.

help researchers contact him, and finally the fathers had to agree to participate. Mothers were asked about men other than the child's biological father only if they reported that the biological father did not reside in the home. If the biological father was not living with the child, mothers were asked about both the biological father and other men who might be like a father to the child. Our specific research questions were as follows: (1) What is the relation between classes of father connectedness and child outcomes? and (2) Are these relations consistent across racial and ethnic groups?

METHODS

Sample

The sample consisted of all mothers who were interviewed when their focus child was about 36 months old and at least one other point (when the child was either 14 or 24 months old), and for whom there were associated assessments of the focus child at 36 months ($N = 1{,}930$). Sample sizes for individual variables and for regression models vary as a result of missing child outcomes data, with the high end for the aggressive behavior outcome (*ns* = 1,284–1,832). The wide range of sample sizes across outcomes is the result of data collection methods. There were fewer child assessments than parent interviews and all child outcomes with the exception of aggressiveness were obtained from in-home child assessments. To retain maximum sample, we imputed missing control variables after determining that those missing on control variables did not differ from the rest of the sample. We did this by running regressions for all the child outcomes using control variables with missing values set to zero and including dummy indicators of "missingness" for each variable. We found no significant relations for these indicators.

Procedures

Classification of father connectedness. Study children were grouped based on our understanding of theory and hypotheses about the importance of different aspects of the father – child relationship into five classes of father connectedness. These classes took into account three dimensions: (1) the degree of biological and social relatedness to the child; (2) residential status vis-à-vis the child's mother or, if nonresident, the frequency with which he saw the child; and (3) a measure of stability (or lack thereof) of these relationships. We combined information from mothers' reports over time to identify stable versus unstable relationships. The classes represented a rough continuum ranging from a child living constantly with the biological father to a child with no or infrequent contact with the biological father and no relationship with a father figure. We formed four classes that represented various types of stable relationships and one class of unstable relationship. (Table 2 provides summary descriptions of each class of connectedness.)

We were constrained by the interview content to define father presence in the following ways: a biological father was present if he (1) lived with the child, or (2) was nonresident but saw the child a few times a month or more in the 3 months prior to each completed interview. Father figures (or men who were not the biological father of the child) were present if the mother identified them to be "like a father" to the child. We included stability over time by considering the father's presence reported by the mother at each interview. Classes are listed in descending order of their hypothesized connectedness to the child's life.

Class 1 is "Stable Resident Biological Father," which indicates that mothers reported, at each completed interview, that the child lived with the biological father "all or part of the time."

Class 2 refers to "Nonresident Involved Biological Fathers." These men either lived with the child sporadically or never lived with the child but saw the child at least a few times a month. We considered this group to represent a form of stability, because it included some men who had lived with the child at the time of one or more interviews and who maintained a consistent presence in the child's life, despite not having been continuously in residence. We tested models that separated biological fathers who were sporadically resident and nonresident, and those who were consistently nonresident (each seeing the child at least at the required frequency), but found there were no differences between the groups relative to the outcomes. Therefore, for parsimony, we combined the groups.

Class 3, termed "Stable Father Figure," included children whose biological fathers saw them less than a few times a month but who had a father figure at the time of each completed interview. We constrained this group to include only children whose mothers reported the same man as the father figure at each interview. This class included the most diverse group of men, ranging from the mothers' current romantic partners to relatives (such as grandfathers) not living with them.

Class 4 is "No Father Presence," which includes children whose biological fathers saw them less than a few times a month in the 3 months prior to each completed interview and for whom there was no other man who functioned like a father to them.

TABLE 2
Definitions of Male Presence by Mother Report Across Two or More Periods

Classes of Father Presence	Definition — Mothers' Report	*N*
Class 1: Stable resident biological father	Resident biological father — Yes Stable — Yes	746
Class 2: Nonresident involved biological father	Resident biological father — Yes (*n* = 216) — No, but sees the child a few times a month or more (*n* = 200) Stable — Yes	416
Class 3: Stable father figure	Resident biological father — No, and sees child less than a few times a month Father figure — Yes Stable — Yes	104
Class 4: No father presence	Resident biological father — No and sees child less than a few times a month Father figure — No Stable — Yes	74
Class 5: Unstable father presence	Combination of these (in any order) Nonresident biological father and father figure (*n* = 145) Nonresident biological father and no father presence (*n* = 111) Father figure and no father presence (*n* = 142) Any other combination (*n* = 200)	590

Note. We defined "stable" relationships as follows. Class 1 resident biological fathers were stable because mothers reported that the biological fathers lived with the child at all interviews. Class 2 fathers were stable because this group included men whose residence had changed according to the mothers but who had remained in close contact with their child, regardless of residency. Mothers were asked about father figures if the biological father was nonresident. In Class 3, if the mother reported on a father figure, he was considered to be stable if she reported on the same man at each interview. (Only children whose nonresident biological fathers did not see them at least a few times a month were placed into Class 3.) Class 4, the "no father presence" group, was stable because there was never any reported father presence at the levels we defined at any interview point. Class 5 was unstable because frequency of seeing the child varied over time.

Class 5 is "Unstable Father Presence," which consisted of all other combinations of resident or nonresident biological father, father figure, or no father presence over all completed interview periods that were not defined by classes 1, 2, 3, or 4. Children in Class 5 had fathers or father figures who fell into different classes at each interview period. On the whole, these children had no stability in father involvement and an absence of the biological father at 36 months; therefore, they were placed into Class 5. We selected Class 5 as the reference group because it represented what appeared to include the most heterogeneous mix of biological and nonbiological relationships combined with tenuousness and inconstancy relative to the other classes. We hypothesized that this class represented the least desirable situation for children in that changes in key parenting figures and gaps in relationships tend to create stress and reduce the likelihood of developing positive social skills and forming supportive social networks (McLanahan & Bumpass, 1988). Therefore, all regression models contained 4 classes (Classes 1 through 4, omitting Class 5) with coefficients interpreted relative to the unstable father class.

Child outcomes. As noted in the introductory article in this Special Issue, trained field staff also conducted a battery of child assessments at the time of the 36-month parent interviews. We selected a range of these outcomes to represent all the major developmental domains: (1) socioemotional, (2) language, (3) cognitive, and (4) behavioral problems. The measure of cognitive development was the Bayley Mental Development Index (MDI; Amato, Keith, & Bayley, 1993). The measures of language development were the Peabody Picture Vocabulary Test – III (PPVT – III; Dunn & Dunn, 1997) and the Test de Vocabulario en Imagenes Peabody (TVIP; Dunn, Padilla, Lugo, & Dunn, 1986). Socioemotional development was assessed using two scales from the Bayley Behavior Rating Scale — Self Regulation and Orientation (Amato et al., 1993). Problem behaviors were derived from the Aggressive Behavior subscale of the Childhood Behavior Checklist (Achenbach & Rescorla, 2000). These are all widely used measures with high levels of reliability and validity, both in their norming samples and for the Early Head Start sample (Administration for Children and Families, 2002).

Control variables. We selected control variables that were of theoretical importance to children's developmental outcomes, to paternal behavior, or to both. The control variables included in our overall equations encompassed primarily characteristics measured at baseline, as well as a few that were measured at 36 months: (1) program status (because Early Head Start participation had a significant effect on some of the outcomes we consider); (2) family demographics: mothers' race (including only European American, African American, and Latin American categories), mothers' education, whether the mother was a teen at the birth of the focus child, urban residence, and welfare receipt; (3) maternal stress: the 36-month Parenting Distress (PD) subscale from the Parenting Stress Index (PSI; Abidin, 1995); (4) quality of parent – child relationships: the 36-month Parent –

Child Dysfunctional Interaction (PCDI) from the PSI; and (5) child gender. Both the PD and the PCDI were used, because they represented ephemeral stressful emotional states that were likely to vary over time (Abidin, 1995). Table 1 shows means of the sample characteristics used as control variables for the overall sample and within race and ethnicity subgroups.

Analytic Approach

To answer the first research question, "What is the relation between levels of father presence and child outcomes?" we regressed each of the child outcome measures on classes of father connectedness (dummy-coded with "unstable father" presence as the reference class), and control variables. To answer the second research question, "Do these relations differ across racial and ethnic groups?" we regressed each child outcome measure on the models described earlier but expanded them to include interactions between race and ethnicity (dummy-coded with European Americans as the reference group) and each class of father presence. We estimated these interacted models including dummies for race and ethnicity to test whether the classes of father presence jointly differed by race and ethnicity. The *F* test of this model indicated that there were such differences on several outcomes across racial and ethnic groups. Therefore, we estimated separate models for each of the three racial and ethnic groups using the same models described earlier.

RESULTS

Table 3 displays regression results for the full sample. The model regressed each child outcome on the various classes of father connectedness (Class 5, "unstable father," was the reference class), and control variables (program status, family demographics, treatment group status, maternal stress, parent–child relationship quality, and child gender). All father connectedness coefficients should be interpreted in terms of their relation to the dependent child outcome relative to the unstable father presence (Class 5) group. Table 4 displays regression results for each of the three major racial and ethnic groups separately.

Full Sample

Family demographic characteristics and parent – child relationship quality variables were related to child outcome measures in expected ways (Table 3). Minority children generally had lower scores on cognitive, lan-

TABLE 3

Regressing Child Developmental Outcomes on Father Presence, Entire Sample

	Child Developmental Outcome									
	Orientation - Engagement		Self-Regulation		PPVT-III		Bayley MDI		CBCL Aggressive	
Regressors	*B*	*SE*	*B*	*SE*	*B*	*SE*	*B*	*SE*	*B*	*SE*
Father class										
Stable resident biological father	–0.05	0.05	0.11*	0.05	0.36	1.07	0.35	0.81	–1.16**	0.35
Nonresident biological father	0.02	0.05	0.11*	0.05	1.50	1.08	0.93	0.86	–1.07**	0.38
Stable father figure	–0.15	0.08	–0.17	0.09	–1.41	1.84	–0.60	1.51	–0.10	0.63
No father presence	0.01	0.09	0.07	0.10	2.32	2.30	1.57	1.64	0.47	0.74
EHS program group	0.04	0.03	0.04	0.04	1.90*	0.81	1.63**	0.62	–0.40	0.27
Race and ethnicity										
African American	–0.33***	0.04	0.05	0.05	–6.84***	0.95	–6.84***	0.77	–1.26***	0.34
Latin American	–0.41***	0.05	–0.02	0.05	–9.20***	1.31	–4.01***	0.84	–0.89*	0.38
Mother's education (years)										
12 years or GED	0.10*	0.04	0.03	0.05	1.98	1.05	2.89***	0.80	0.91*	0.35
More than 12 years	0.26***	0.05	0.22***	0.05	7.86***	1.17	5.31***	0.89	0.60	0.39
Teen mother at birth of focus child	0.17***	0.04	0.04	0.05	–0.03	0.98	0.66	0.74	0.16	0.33
Family lives in urban area	0.30***	0.04	–0.06	0.04	3.87***	0.85	2.84***	0.64	–0.19	0.28
Family received welfare	–0.05	0.04	–0.08	0.04	–1.57	0.86	–1.12	0.66	–0.05	0.29
Parent - child dysfunctional interaction	0.00	0.00	–0.01**	0.00	–0.28***	0.08	–0.24***	0.06	0.32***	0.03
Parenting distress	0.00*	0.00	0.00	0.00	–0.08	0.05	–0.03	0.04	0.12***	0.02
Boy	–0.09**	0.03	–0.26***	0.04	–3.01***	0.81	–2.00**	0.62	0.94***	0.27
N	1,591		1,583		1,284		1,491		1,832	

Note. PPVT - III = Peabody Picture Vocabulary Test-Third Edition; MDI = Mental Development Index; CBCL = Child Behavior Checklist; GED = government equivalency diploma.

*$p < .05$. **$p < .01$. ***$p < .001$.

TABLE 4
Regressing Child Developmental Outcomes on Father Presence Within Race and Ethnicity

	Child Developmental Outcomes									
	Orientation - Engagement		Self-Regulation		PPVT-III		Bayley MDI		Bayley MDI	
	B	*SE*	*B*	*SE*	*B*	*SE*	*B*	*SE*	*B*	*SE*
European American										
Father class										
Stable resident biological father	–0.03	0.07	0.22**	0.08	0.14	1.53	2.48*	1.25	–1.33*	0.53
Nonresident biological father	–0.07	0.08	0.17	0.09	2.16	1.83	1.44	1.49	–1.32*	0.64
Stable father figure	–0.27*	0.11	–0.09	0.13	–2.10	2.56	–0.18	2.17	0.45	0.87
No father presence	0.20	0.15	0.14	0.17	6.11	3.39	4.94	2.82	–0.40	1.22
EHS program group	–0.02	0.05	–0.01	0.06	1.37	1.20	1.83	0.99	–0.06	0.41
Mother's education (years)										
12 years or GED	0.05	0.07	0.15	0.08	0.90	1.53	2.30	1.25	0.58	0.54
More than 12 years	0.24**	0.08	0.35***	0.08	9.45***	1.70	7.89***	1.40	0.75	0.60
Teen mother at birth of focus child	0.11	0.06	0.03	0.07	0.74	1.47	1.26	1.20	–0.28	0.52
Family lives in urban area	0.07	0.06	–0.12	0.06	–0.27	1.27	–1.65	1.04	–0.42	0.43
Family received welfare	–0.12*	0.06	–0.04	0.06	–0.88	1.28	–0.47	1.06	0.09	0.44
Parent - child dysfunctional interaction	–0.02**	0.01	–0.03***	0.01	–0.54***	0.13	–0.36***	0.11	0.40***	0.04
Parenting distress	0.00	0.00	0.01**	0.00	0.03	0.08	0.04	0.06	0.15	0.03
Boy	–0.09	0.05	–0.41***	0.06	–3.95***	1.20	–2.11*	0.99	1.21**	0.41
N	621		618		589		578		711	

(continued)

TABLE 4 *(Continued)*

	Child Developmental Outcomes									
	Orientation - Engagement		Self-Regulation		PPVT-III		Bayley MDI		Bayley MDI	
	B	*SE*	*B*	*SE*	*B*	*SE*	*B*	*SE*	*B*	*SE*
African American Regressors										
Father class										
Stable resident biological father	–0.16	0.09	–0.12	0.10	–1.87	1.83	–3.32*	1.52	–1.78*	0.70
Nonresident biological father	0.03	0.07	0.01	0.08	0.52	1.43	0.46	1.18	–1.01	0.54
Stable father figure	0.08	0.15	–0.22	0.17	1.25	3.11	2.44	2.72	–0.56	1.14
No father presence	0.06	0.15	–0.03	0.17	–2.53	3.26	–2.36	2.59	1.22	1.14
EHS program group	0.07	0.06	0.09	0.07	2.51*	1.22	1.14	1.02	–1.28**	0.46
Mother's education (years)										
12 years or GED	0.06	0.08	–0.08	0.09	2.94	1.64	5.45***	1.37	1.11	0.62
More than 12 years	0.22*	0.09	0.03	0.10	4.08*	1.88	4.61**	1.57	0.87	0.72
Teen mother at birth of focus child	0.19*	0.07	0.01	0.08	–0.62	1.51	1.65	1.26	0.31	0.58
Family lives in urban area	0.53***	0.06	–0.10	0.07	7.41***	1.29	9.28***	1.07	1.08*	0.49
Family received welfare	–0.01	0.06	–0.08	0.07	–2.76*	1.32	–1.12	1.09	0.35	0.50
Parent - child dysfunctional interaction	0.00	0.01	–0.02**	0.01	–0.05	0.11	–0.15	0.09	0.34***	0.04
Parenting distress	–0.01	0.00	0.00	0.00	–0.11	0.07	–0.01	0.06	0.08**	0.03
Boy	–0.14*	0.06	–0.13*	0.07	–2.11	1.23	–2.27*	1.01	0.37	0.46
N	516		515		475		482		608	

	Orientation - Engagement		Self-Regulation		PPVT-III		TVIP		Bayley MDI		CBCL Aggressive	
	B	*SE*	*B*	*SE*	*B*	*SE*	B	*SE*	*B*	*SE*	*B*	*SE*
Latin American Regressors												
Father class												
Stable resident biological father	–0.05	0.10	0.18	0.10	6.49*	3.20	0.41	1.60	–1.07	1.62	–0.79	0.81
Nonresident biological father	0.37**	0.13	0.23	0.13	6.30	3.24	–1.29	3.38	5.34*	2.10	–0.80	1.07
Stable father figure	–0.14	0.21	–0.40	0.22	0.07	6.41	–0.43	4.69	–3.62	3.51	–1.04	1.76
No father presence	–0.11	0.19	0.26	0.20	10.19	9.54	0.85	2.50	2.89	3.09	0.33	1.68
EHS program group	0.09	0.08	0.03	0.08	1.50	2.57	1.30	1.10	2.42*	1.23	0.05	0.63
Mother's education (years)												
12 years or GED	0.11	0.11	0.05	0.11	4.12	3.27	1.08	1.87	0.63	1.78	0.96	0.90
More than 12 years	0.22	0.11	0.15	0.12	12.42***	3.56	1.05	1.70	1.43	1.86	0.41	0.99
Teen mother at birth of focus child	0.16	0.09	0.08	0.09	–2.10	2.84	–0.84	1.46	–2.64	1.41	0.59	0.73
Family lives in urban area	0.44***	0.08	0.17*	0.09	11.25***	2.90	4.16***	1.24	4.13**	1.34	–1.46*	0.70
Family received welfare	–0.01	0.08	–0.06	0.09	–0.28	2.84	–2.48*	1.22	–3.13*	1.35	–1.24	0.69
Parent - child dysfunctional interaction	0.01	0.01	0.00	0.01	–0.38	0.26	–0.03	0.08	–0.22*	0.10	0.23***	0.05
Parenting distress	–0.01	0.00	0.00	0.00	0.01	0.15	–0.07	0.06	–0.06	0.07	0.11**	0.04
Boy	–0.02	0.07	–0.17*	0.08	–0.67	2.54	–0.68	1.07	–0.96	1.22	0.99	0.63
N	391		387		164		208		371		433	

Note. PPVT - III = Peabody Picture Vocabulary Test-Third Edition; TVIP = Test de Vocabularie en Imagenes Peabody; MDI = Mental Development Index; CBCL = Child Behavior Checklist; GED = government equivalency diploma.

*$p < .05$. **$p < .01$. ***$p < .001$.

guage, and socioemotional measures but were not different from European American children in self-regulation. As expected, maternal education was positively related to child outcomes, particularly in the cognitive domain (Bradley & Corwyn, 2002). Boys scored lower than girls on cognitive and regulatory domains and higher on aggression. Dysfunctional parent – child interactions were associated with poorer outcomes in most domains, but living in an urban area, having a teenage mother, and experiencing parenting distress had mixed relations to child outcomes.

Important for this study, we found significant relations between classes of father connectedness and two key child outcomes — self-regulation and aggression. We present effect sizes for ease of comparison across findings. Effect sizes (ES) were calculated by dividing regression coefficients by the standard deviation of the outcome variable then multiplying by 100 (interpreted as a percentage of a standard deviation), p values refer to the significance of the coefficient in the regression model. Children in the "nonresident biological father" class, $ES = 13.8, p < .05$, and the "resident biological father" class, $ES = 14.3, p < .05$, showed higher levels of self-regulation than children in the "unstable father" class, and they were also less aggressive ($ES = 16.6, p < .01$, and $ES = 18.0, p < .01$, for "nonresident" and "resident biological father" classes, respectively). There were no significant relations between the classes of father connectedness and any of the other child outcomes examined.

To answer the second research question, we tested whether the relation between the explanatory variables and outcomes varied across racial and ethnic groups. First, we estimated the regression models described for the entire sample and included interactions between racial and ethnic group status and father connectedness classes. In several cases, the father presence and race interaction terms were statistically significant, which indicates that the relation between the presence of a father and a particular child outcome varied by race. We found significant relations between interaction terms and these outcomes: orientation and engagement (Latin American nonresident biological father, $p < .01$); self-regulation (African American resident biological father, $p < .01$); PPVT – III (Latin American biological father, $p < .05$); and MDI (African American resident biological father, $p < .01$). Given the significance of these interaction terms, we examined relations between father connectedness and the child outcomes within race and ethnicity. Specifically, we reran the regression models displayed in Table 3 for European Americans, African Americans, and Latin Americans separately, omitting the dummy-coded race and ethnicity variables in the models. These models are displayed in Table 4. In general, we found that classes of father connectedness function differently by sociocultural group with respect to these child outcomes

European Americans

For European Americans, the relation between family demographic variables and child outcomes were in the expected direction, with maternal education correlated with the greatest number of outcomes. In addition, higher quality parent – child relationships were associated with better outcomes, also as expected. In general, parenting distress was not significant in the models, except in the case of self-regulation and aggressiveness, where high maternal distress was associated with lower self-regulation and higher child aggressiveness. Urban residence had little relation to child outcomes.

Compared with children from the "unstable father" reference group, children in the "father figure" group, $ES = 36.6, p < .05$, showed lower levels of orientation and engagement. We found positive relations between classes of father connectedness and cognitive performance, on the MDI — children with resident biological fathers performed better than those in the omitted group, $ES = 19.6, p < .05$. There were no differences in self regulation, language, or aggressiveness.

African Americans

Among African Americans, relations between family demographic variables and child outcomes were generally consistent with expectations. Parent – child dysfunctional interactions were positively correlated with behavior problems. Parenting distress also was associated with child aggressiveness, but the association was weaker, $ES = .10, p < .01$. Urban residence was positively associated with five of six outcomes.

The significant associations between the classes of father connectedness and child outcomes were mixed. There were no relations between father connectedness and self-regulation. African American children in nonresident biological father classes showed lower levels of aggression, $ES = 15.6$, $p < .05$. Living with a biological father was associated with poorer MDI scores, $ES = 26.3, p <. 05$, relative to the "unstable father" group.

Latin Americans

Results for Latin Americans revealed few relations between most control variables and child outcomes. Even maternal education and quality of parent – child relationships were related to only a few child outcome measures. The most consistent positive relation was between living in an urban area and each of the outcomes. Regarding father connectedness, children in both biological-father-presence classes had higher scores on the PPVT –

III relative to the "unstable father" group, $ES = 40.5, p < .01$, and $ES = 41.7, p < .05$, for nonresident and resident biological groups, respectively. However, there were no significant relations to the TVIP and sample sizes for both measures are small. Latin American children in the "nonresident biological father" group performed better on the MDI, $ES = 42.2, p < .05$, and had better orientation and engagement, $ES = 50.9, p < .01$, than children in the "unstable father" group.

DISCUSSION

Overall, our findings suggest a complex relation between classes of father presence and child developmental outcomes. To some degree, children living with their biological fathers seem developmentally better off, primarily in the self-regulatory and behavioral domains. The findings are consistent with those reported in this Special Issue by Fitzgerald, McKelvey, Schiffman, and Montanez, suggesting that fathers may be particularly important for helping very young children gain control over intense emotions. Although mothers tend to spend more time with their children, their encounters include more verbal interactions, whereas fathers' are more physical (Parke, 1995) and may both stimulate and help to regulate strong feelings. In our models, maternal education likely absorbs much of the family variation in maternal talk and engagement in learning activities. Because of assortive mating, maternal education may also absorb part of the variation in father talk and engagement in learning activities with children, consistent with Tamis-LeMonda, Shannon, Cabrera, and Lamb (2004), who found similarities in parenting behaviors between low-income fathers and mothers. These researchers also found contributions to children's cognitive development, but these contributions were related to the quality of interactions during play, an aspect of father connectedness not measured in this study.

When we considered models within race, however, these relations seemed most straightforward for European Americans. Specifically, among European Americans, a greater and more consistent biological father presence was associated with positive developmental child outcomes. Children with nonresident biological fathers who were at least somewhat involved were better off than those with unstable and transient relationships to their fathers. However, these relations did not hold as consistently for African Americans in the sample. There were some negative and some positive associations, and these did not occur in any pattern that is easily interpretable. Taken as a whole, the results suggest that neither biological relatedness nor family configuration in and of themselves are predictive of what children experience or of the degree to which such relatedness or configuration matters in their development. The likely impact of biological relatedness and family configuration appears to depend on the socioeconomic, political, and cultural niche of family life (Harkness & Super, 2002). These broader aspects of context may create compensatory (e.g., extended family supports) or interfering conditions that reduce the impact of father connectedness or change its valence (Garcia Coll & Pachter, 2002).

The reason for the negative findings among African American resident biological fathers remains unclear. Some research on African American fathers suggests that they are less involved with their children and families than other men (Black, Dubowitz, & Starr, 1999; Crockett, Eggebeen, & Hawkins, 1993). It is also possible that nonresident men present in the lives of African American children were more positive influences on development than the men of other racial and ethnic groups studied, such that contrasts between categories of father connectedness were less pronounced.

The lack of relation between outcomes and most control variables for Latin Americans suggests the need for greater complexity in defining and measuring meaningful background characteristics. For example, the findings pertaining to maternal education may reflect the fact that the sample included many Latin American immigrants, and it is hard to equate educational status for immigrants and nonimmigrants (Fuligni & Yoshikawa, 2003). The strong relations between outcomes and urban residence require further study to determine whether urban residence is associated with other factors that may contribute to developmental success, such as proximity of extended family or nonmigrant status. Indeed, the employment circumstances of many recently immigrated Latin Americans can compromise the level and type of involvement they have with their children even when they reside in the same household.

Limitations

We were able to assess roughly the relations between father connectedness and child outcomes but were unable to measure the quality of the father – child relationship. There is substantial diversity in fathers' roles with their children and within the family than there tends to be for mothers. Mothers typically act as the child's primary caregiver, whereas fathers vary more widely in terms of their caregiving, and tend to spend greater amounts of time in play and physical activities with the child (Horn, 2000). Thus, it is harder to pinpoint the mechanisms by which fathers may influence their children's well-being (Parke, 1995). Although the benefits of father involvement in children's lives may well depend on the quality of the overall relationships within the family and how well the father fits into the overall functioning of the family (Lamb, 1997), a study by Furstenberg and Harris (1993) found little impact of paternal contact alone for African American adolescents but clear evidence that relationship quality made a difference.

Second, for low-income families in particular, the effects of fathers on children may be overwhelmed by elements (for good or ill) that enter family life (Bradley & Corwyn, 2002; Garcia Coll & Pachter, 2002). African American and Latin American families are likely to be low-income and may contain environmental, cultural, or social elements that undermine the father's involvement in children's lives. These elements include greater likelihood of family instability and chronic stress and less consistent access to supportive resources, all of which may have direct negative impacts on children and reduce the likelihood of productive coparenting. McAdoo (2002) made specific reference to the marginalization of African American men and the high levels of family dissolution in African American families. Third, especially in the case of Latin American children, developmental outcomes may be measured with less validity than is the case for European American children.

Last, our sample of low-income families does not generalize to all low-income families. Our sample is a select one, consisting of families who were interested in participating in a study of Early Head Start, participated in lengthy interviews, and allowed assessments of their child. Although we cannot generalize to all low-income families, we feel confident that findings from this study add to the literature on what fathering means for low-income families. Consistent with the broader literature on paternal residence status, findings from this study show sociocultural group differences in the likelihood that fathers will live with a child and spend significant amounts of time with a child. For example, European American and Latin American children are more likely to have a resident biological father than African Americans. It will be important to examine how relations between father – child connectedness and child outcomes change over time within racial and ethnic groups.

Next Steps

As children grow and the "match" between their activities converges, fathers tend to increase the time they spend as their child's playmate (Fitzgerald & McKelvey, 2005). If father – child contact increases, we may then expect bigger influences with time. However, if children have little stability in their relationships with fathers and father figures, then there is little reason to expect cumulative influences. Moreover, if there is the anticipation of low stability, there may be lower likelihood of synchronized, supportive parenting actions within the family or from extended family (e.g., the kind of redundancy within systems that leads to stronger effects). We begin to examine these issues by using data collected about the Early Head Start children just before they enter kindergarten.

Future research should also examine how resident biological fathers could be divided into those who are involved with the children's mothers in romantic relationships that involve a long-term commitment versus those who are not. Furthermore, it would be useful to examine whether and how these relationships differ across racial and ethnic groups.

It will also be useful to examine the indirect effects of levels of father presence on child outcomes. For example, the Fragile Families and Child Wellbeing Study observed positive associations between father involvement and maternal health and children's outcomes in terms of fewer lower birthweight deliveries. Using Early Head Start data, we can examine whether father presence (or particular father behaviors) mitigates negative mother characteristics (for example, by lessening the negative effect of mothers' depression; Kahn, Brandt, & Whitacker, 2004) or exacerbates poor home situations (for example, by augmenting the negative effect of mothers' depression). We could also examine whether the stable committed presence of fathers in children's lives enhances the positive behavior of mothers (e.g., provides support or redundancy leading to greater impact). Better understanding of these family systems effects can aid programs like Early Head Start in developing targeted and individualized services for families.

AFFILIATIONS AND ADDRESSES

Cheri A. Vogel, Mathematica Policy Research, Inc., 600 Alexander Park, Princeton, NJ 08540. E-mail: cvogel@mathematica-mpr.com. Robert H. Bradley is at the University of Arkansas at Little Rock. Helen H. Raikes is at the University of Nebraska–Lincoln and the Gallup Organization. Kimberly Boller is also at Mathematica Policy Research, Inc. Jeffrey K. Shears is at Colorado State University.

ACKNOWLEDGMENTS

We gratefully acknowledge the contributions of Ece Kalay for the variable construction and SAS programming that made this work possible. We are also indebted to Judy Carta and Mark Fine, who reviewed earlier drafts of the article. Jill Constantine provided valuable technical assistance and advice in developing our models. Laura Hawkinson assisted us with the literature review and Bryan Gustus formatted the document. Any errors that remain are our own. The content of this publication does not necessarily reflect the views or policies of the Department of Health and Human Services, and mention of trade names, commercial products, or organizations does not imply endorsement by the U.S. Government.

REFERENCES

Abidin, R. R. (1995). *Parenting Stress Index* (3rd ed.). Odessa, FL: Psychological Assessment Resources.

Achenbach, T. M., & Rescorla, L. A. (2000). *Manual for the ASEBA Preschool Forms and Profiles.* Burlington: University of Vermont Department of Psychiatry.

Administration for Children & Families. (2002). *Pathways to quality and full implementation in Early Head Start programs.* Washington, DC: Department of Health and Human Services.

Amato, P. R. (1993). Contact with non-custodial fathers and children's wellbeing. *Family Matters, 36,* 32–34.

Amato, P. R., & Keith, B. (1991). Separation from a parent during childhood and adult socioeconomic attainment. *Social Forces, 70,* 187–206.

Amato, P. R., Keith, B., & Bayley, N. (1993). *Bayley Scales of Infant Development, second edition: Manual.* New York: Psychological Corporation.

Biller, H. B. (1982). Fatherhood: Implications for child and adult development. In B. B. Wolman & G. Stricker (Eds.), *Handbook of developmental psychology* (pp. 702–725). Englewood Cliffs, NJ: Prentice Hall.

Black, M. M., Dubowitz, H., & Starr, R. H. (1999). African American fathers in low-income, urban families: Development, behavior, and home environment of their three year old children. *Child Development, 70,* 967–978.

Blankenhorn, D. G., Jr. (1995). *Fatherless America: Confronting our most urgent social problem.* New York: Basic Books.

Bradley, R. H., & Corwyn, R. F. (2002). SES and child development. *Annual Review of Psychology, 53,* 371–399.

Cabrera, N. J., Tamis-LeMonda, C. S., Bradley, R. H., Hofferth, S., & Lamb, M. E. (2000). Fatherhood in the twenty-first century. *Child Development, 71,* 127–137.

Crockett, L. J., Eggebeen, D. J., & Hawkins, A. J. (1993). Father's presence and young children's behavioral and cognitive adjustment. *Journal of Family Issues, 14,* 355–377.

Curran L., & Abrams L. S. (2000). Making men into dads: Fatherhood, the state, and welfare reform. *Gender & Society, 14,* 662–678.

Dunn, L. M., & Dunn, L. M. (1997). *Peabody Picture Vocabulary Test–Third Edition.* Circle Pines, MN: American Guidance Service.

Dunn, L. M., Padilla, E. R., Lugo, D. E., & Dunn, L. M. (1986). *Examiner's Manual for the Test de Vocabulario en Imagenes Peabody. Adaptacion Hispanoamericana.* Circle Pines, MN: American Guidance Service.

England, P., & Folbre, N. (2002). Involving dads: Parental bargaining and family well-being. In C. S. Tamis-LeMonda & N. Cabrera (Eds.), *Handbook of father involvement: Multidisciplinary perspectives* (pp. 387–408). Mahwah, NJ: Lawrence Erlbaum Associates, Inc.

Fitzgerald, H. E., & McKelvey, L. M. (2005). Low-income adolescent fathers: Risk for parenthood and risky parenting. *Zero to Three, 25*(4), 35–41.

Furstenberg, F. F., & Harris, K. M. (1993). When and why fathers matter: Impacts of father involvement on children of adolescent mothers. In R. I. Lehman & T. J. Ooms (Eds.), *Young unwed fathers* (pp. 117–138). Philadelphia: Temple University Press.

Fuligni, A. J., & Yoshikawa, H. (2003). Socioeconomic resources, parenting, and child development among immigrant families. In M. Bornstein & R. Bradley (Eds.), *Socioeconomic status, parenting, and child deveopment* (pp. 107–124). Mahwah, NJ: Lawrence Erlbaum Associates, Inc.

Garcia Coll, C., & Pachter, L. M. (2002). Ethnic and minority parenting. In M. H. Bornstein (Ed.), *Handbook of parenting, Vol. 4: Social condition and applied parenting* (2nd ed., pp. 1–20). Mahwah, NJ: Lawrence Erlbaum Associates, Inc.

Graham, J. W., & Beller, A. H. (2002). Nonresident fathers and their children: Child support and visitation from an economic perspective. In C. S. Tamis-LeMonda & N. Cabrera (Eds.), *Handbook of father involvement* (pp 33–64). Mahwah, NJ: Lawrence Erlbaum Associates, Inc.

Harkness, S., & Super, C. M. (2002). Culture and parenting. In M. Bornstein (Ed.), *Handbook of parenting, Vol. 4: Social conditions and applied parenting* (2nd ed., pp. 253–280). Mahwah, NJ: Lawrence Erlbaum Associates, Inc.

Hines, A. M. (1997). Divorce-related transitions, adolescent development, and the role of the parent–child relationship: A review of the literature. *Journal of Marriage and the Family, 59,* 375–388.

Hofferth, S. L. (1984). Kin networks, race, and family structure. *Journal of Marriage and the Family, 46,* 791–806.

Horn, W. F. (2000). Fathering infants. In J. Osofsky & H. Fitzgerald (Eds.), *WAIMH handbook of infant mental health, volume III* (pp. 272–298). New York: Wiley.

Kahn, R. S., Brandt, D., & Whitaker, R. C. (2004). Combined effects of mothers' and fathers' mental health symptoms on children's behavioral and emotional well-being. *Pediatric and Adolescent Medicine, 158*(8), 721–729.

Lamb, M. E. (1997). Fathers and child development: An introductory overview. In M. E. Lamb (Ed.), *The role of the father in child development* (3rd ed., pp. 1–18). New York: Wiley.

Lamb, M. E. (2002). Infant–father attachments and their impact on child development. In C. S. Tamis-LeMonda & N. Cabrera (Eds.), *Handbook of father involvement* (pp. 33–64). Mahwah, NJ: Lawrence Erlbaum Associates, Inc.

McAdoo, H. P. (2002). African American parenting. In M. H. Bornstein (Ed.), *Handbook of parenting, Vol. 4: Social conditions and applied parenting* (2nd ed., pp. 47–58). Mahwah, NJ: Lawrence Erlbaum Associates, Inc.

McLanahan, S., & Bumpass, L. (1988). Intergenerational consequences of family disruption. *American Journal of Sociology, 94,* 130–152.

Palkovitz, R. (2002). Involved fathering and child development: Advancing our understanding of good fathering. In C. S. Tamis-LeMonda & N. Cabrera (Eds.), *Handbook of father involvement* (pp. 119–140). Mahwah, NJ: Lawrence Erlbaum Associates, Inc.

Parke, R. D. (1995). Fathers and families. In M. H. Bornstein (Ed.), *Handbook of parenting, Vol. 3: Status and social conditions of parenting* (2nd ed., pp. 27–74). Mahwah, NJ: Lawrence Erlbaum Associates, Inc.

Pollack, R. A., & Ginther, D. K. (2003, April). *Does family structure affect children's educational outcomes?* (Working Paper no. 9628). Cambridge, MA: National Bureau of Economic Research.

Tamis-LeMonda, C., Shannon, J., Cabrera, N., & Lamb, M. (2004). Fathers and mothers at play with their 2- and 3-year olds; contributions to language and cognitive development. *Child Development, 75*(6), 1806–1820.

PARENTING: SCIENCE AND PRACTICE April–September 2006 Volume 6 Numbers 2 & 3 Pages 211–228

Is One Good Parent Good Enough? Patterns of Mother and Father Parenting and Child Cognitive Outcomes at 24 and 36 Months

Rebecca M. Ryan, Anne Martin, and Jeanne Brooks-Gunn

SYNOPSIS

Objective. This study examined parenting patterns in a sample of low-income couples and the impact of those patterns on young children's cognitive outcomes. ***Design.*** Interactions between 237 mothers, fathers, and their 2-year-old children were examined among coresident mothers and fathers or father figures who participated in the Early Head Start Research and Evaluation Project's Father and Child Interaction During Toddlerhood Study (FACITS). Scores on 6 parenting scales were entered into K-means cluster analyses to determine whether different parenting patterns emerged by gender. Analyses of covariance were used to examine how the behavior of each parent alone and both parents jointly was associated with child cognitive outcomes concurrently and 1 year later. ***Results.*** Mothers and fathers exhibited similar parenting patterns, with Highly Supportive (43% of mothers, 34% of fathers), Somewhat Supportive (35%, 43%), Detached (8%, 15%), and Negative (14%, 8%) clusters emerging for both genders. However, differences emerged between the Detached and Negative mother and father clusters, with higher detachment among Detached mothers and higher negativity among Negative fathers. For mothers at both time points and fathers at 36 months, children with Highly Supportive parents had higher Bayley Mental Development Index (MDI) scores than children in the 2 non-Supportive clusters, controlling for parent demographics and income. Children with 2 Supportive parents scored higher on the Bayley MDI than all other children, whereas those with no Supportive parents were particularly disadvantaged. Having at least 1 Supportive mother or father benefited children's cognitive development over having none. ***Conclusions.*** Children who have at least 1 Supportive parent score higher on cognitive assessments, regardless of parent gender, than those with none; studies on parenting and child development should consider mother and father behavior in concert.

INTRODUCTION

Countless studies have established the importance of maternal supportiveness to early child cognitive development (see Bornstein, 2002, for a review), with warmth, stimulation, involvement, and responsiveness (or contingency) associated with positive early childhood outcomes (De Wolff & van Ijzendoorn, 1997; Duncan & Brooks-Gunn, 1997; Landry, Smith, Swank, Assel, & Vellet, 2001; National Institute of Child Health and Human Development [NICHD], 1999; Pettit, Bates, & Dodge, 1997; Rothbaum & Weisz, 1994). Although the earliest research on the influence of parenting on early child development focused almost exclusively on mothers, since the 1970s, studies on father parenting have found that men are as capable as women of behaving in sensitive, responsive, nurturing, and stimulating ways with babies and children (Belsky, 1979; Conner, Knight, & Cross, 1997; Lamb, 1997), with some exceptions (Belsky, Gilstrap, & Rovine, 1984; Bentley & Fox, 1991; Power & Parke, 1983; Lamb, Frodi, Hwang, Frodi, & Steinberg, 1982). These studies have also shown that, as with mothers, sensitivity, responsiveness, and stimulation among fathers predict better cognitive outcomes for infants and young children (Black, Dubowitz, & Starr, 1999; Kelley, Smith, Green, Berndt, & Rogers, 1998; Lamb, 1997; Shannon, Tamis-LeMonda, London, & Cabrera, 2002; Tamis-LeMonda, Shannon, Cabrera, & Lamb, 2004; Yogman, Kindlon, & Earls, 1995), even when holding constant the quality of mothers' parenting within the same family (e.g., Shannon et al., 2002; Tamis-LeMonda et al., 2004). It has thus been established that parenting behaviors in mothers and fathers independently influence child development.

This study builds on these efforts by considering combinations of mother and father parenting style. Little attention has been paid to the homogamy of parenting within families and the effects of convergent or divergent parenting behaviors on young children. For example, although it is known that supportive parenting by mothers and fathers independently predicts better developmental outcomes in infants and young children, the consequences of supportive parenting by one parent and nonsupportive parenting by the other have received scant attention (an exception is Elder, 1974). Furthermore, to our knowledge, no studies have explored whether the influence of one parent's parenting style varies according to the parenting style of the other parent. It is possible, for example, that the advantages conferred by one supportive parent can be significantly diminished or even offset by a nonsupportive parent. It is also possible that the benefits of having one supportive parent may be enhanced by having a second supportive parent, for that combination would provide a consistently positive parenting environment. We suggest in particular that a supportive father, who often serves as a secondary caregiver, may augment the advantages of a supportive mother, who is most often the primary caregiver. In testing this hypothesis, we consider the possibility that mother and father parenting styles interact to produce effects that are unidentifiable in studies of mother and father main effects. We also determine the relevance of parent gender to certain parenting combinations.

Before examining the effects of mother and father parenting, we test the appropriateness of applying identical measures of observed parenting style to men and women. With few exceptions (Ban & Lewis, 1974; Bentley & Fox, 1991), studies typically compare mothers and fathers using group means on individual behaviors. Although such efforts demonstrate the utility of applying the same ratings scales to mothers and fathers, it should not be presumed that parenting scales operate similarly across gender. It may be that mothers and fathers can be rated with the same behavior scales, such as those tapping sensitivity or stimulation, but that those scales do not covary among mothers as they do among fathers. For example, mothers who score relatively high on a scale of negative affect may also tend to score relatively high on a scale of positive affect, whereas fathers with relatively high scores on negative affect may not. In such a scenario, mothers may be better described as expressive than negative. Therefore, it is useful to consider variation in mothers' and fathers' parenting styles in addition to particular practices or behaviors. Parenting style, as opposed to discrete parenting behaviors, is conceptualized as a constellation of parenting attitudes and practices that make up an emotional and interactional climate for the child (Darling & Steinberg, 1993).

To identify possible variation in parenting styles, we conduct separate cluster analyses of the same parenting behaviors for mothers and fathers. Cluster analysis is a person-based rather than variable-based approach to quantitative data analysis (Aldenderfer & Blashfield, 1984; Jain & Dubes, 1988) that is well-suited to an inquiry of interactive and nonlinear parenting processes. This method allows us to unveil naturally occurring parenting patterns and reveal differences between those patterns by gender. Based on the clusters that emerge, we classify mothers and fathers separately and then cross-classify them within couples. By measuring mothers' and fathers' parenting styles, rather than individual behaviors, and by considering them jointly, rather than separately, we aim to capture the fullness and complexity of children's actual lived experiences, thus yielding more accurate estimates of the association between children's parenting environment and their cognitive outcomes.

METHODS

Sample

Data were drawn from the Early Head Start Research and Evaluation Project's Father and Child Interaction During Toddlerhood Study (FACITS). For a description of the Early Head Start Father Study and its different strands of data, see Cabrera et al. (2002) and Boller et al. (this issue). Couples included were those mothers and fathers or father figures who were both videotaped with the focus child during the 24-month birthday-related home visit and who lived together at that time ($N = 237$). Only 8 of the 17 Early Head Start research sites collected videotaped data on fathers at 24 months (one video site was eliminated from these analyses because it collected only one videotape); therefore, this sample is drawn only from those sites. Ninety-eight percent ($n = 231$) of participating mothers were the child's biological parent; of the remainder, one was a foster mother, four were grandmothers, and one was another female relative. Eighty-two percent of fathers were biological ($n = 194$), and the other 18% were stepfathers ($n = 21$), grandfathers ($n = 13$), other male relatives ($n = 8$), or foster fathers ($n = 1$). Half of our sample were intervention families ($n = 119$) who had been randomly assigned to receive Early Head Start services, and half were controls ($n = 118$); groups were combined, with program status controlled for in all analyses.

The 237 participating couples made up a diverse low-income sample. Among mothers, 65% were European American, 20% African American, and 12% Latin American, with the remainder of other ethnicities (e.g., American Indian, Asian American); 67% had at least a high school education or government equivalency diploma (GED); and 33% were teenagers (< 20 years old) at the focus child's birth. Among fathers, 60% were European American, 19% African American, and 15% Latin American; 72% had at least a high school education or a GED; and 17% were teenagers at the child's birth. Eighty-two percent of participating couples lived below the federal poverty line at baseline, as would be expected for a sample drawn from Early Head Start, a program that targets low-income families. The mean age of participating children at the time of the mother interview was 25.0 months ($SD = 1.3$); 49% were male and 55% were firstborn.

European Americans were overrepresented in this sample, and African Americans underrepresented when compared to the full videotaped sample of mothers at 24 months because a larger proportion of sites that collected father video data were rural and had more European American participants. In addition, our sample is restricted to coresident couples, who, according to national statistics, are more likely to be European American than African American or Latin American (Padilla & Reichman, 2001; Ventura & Bachrach, 2000). Of the full mother videotaped sample, 39% were European American, 32% African American, 24% Latin American, and 4% other.[1]

Measures

Parenting. Parenting at 24 months was assessed from a 10-min parent–child videotaped interaction. Mothers and fathers were observed separately in dyadic interactions with their child. During the "Three-Bag" task, parents were given intentionally vague instructions regarding the task to elicit naturally occurring individual differences in parenting behaviors (see Boller et al., this issue, for a more thorough description of the procedure). The protocol, adapted from Vandell (1979) and the NICHD Study of Early Child Care (1999) "Three Box" assessment, was used to tap parental sensitivity and insensitivity. Six parenting scales were examined: sensitivity (the extent to which the parent takes the child's perspective, accurately perceives the child's signals, and promptly and appropriately responds to these signals), cognitive stimulation (teaching, actively trying to expand the child's abilities), positive regard (demonstrations of love, respect, and admiration), negative regard (acts of hostility toward or rejection of the child), intrusiveness (physical or verbal overcontrol of the child's play), and detachment (failure to respond to the child's cues for attention, guidance, or affection). All scales were scored on a 7-point range from 1 (*very low*) to 7 (*very high*).[2]

The coding of the Early Head Start 24-month parent–child videotapes was conducted at the National Center for Children and Families, Teachers College, Columbia University, by a team of researchers using scales adapted from the NICHD Study of Early Child Care's "Three Box" scales (Brady-Smith, O'Brien, Berlin, & Ware, 1999; NICHD Early Child Care Research Network, 1999). The coders achieved reliability (exact agreement within 1 point) to a criterion of 85% with the coding team leader, after which 15% of tapes were drawn randomly from the coders' weekly assignment and checked for interrater reliability (again at 85%). Coders' average percentage agreement for parenting scales ranged from 89 to 98 for mother tapes and from 94 to 96 for father tapes. All coders were unaware of the

---

[1]Sample demographic characteristics by cluster are available from the first author on request.

[2]A more thorough description of the Early Head Start 24-Month Parenting Scales is available from the first author on request.

program status and any other identifying information about the videotaped families.

Child outcomes. Child cognitive outcomes at 24 and 36 months were assessed using the Bayley Scales of Infant Development II (BSID – II). The BSID – II is a structured assessment administered to toddlers to measure their mental, motor, and behavioral development. Mental Development Index (MDI) scores reflect performance on the cognitive and language portion of the assessment and parallel other IQ scores with a normed $M = 100$ and $SD = 15$. The mean MDI score for our sample was 92.3 for 24-month-old children and 93.2 for 36-month-old children (SDs = 14.6 and 13.8, respectively). Of the 237 couples, Bayley scores were available for 212 children at 24 months and 196 children at 36 months.

Covariates. Mother race, highest parent education, child gender, and program status were held constant at their means in all analyses of covariance (ANCOVAs). For mothers, this information was taken from data gathered at baseline, prior to random assignment. For fathers, this information was gathered during the 24-month father interview. Maternal race is captured with indicator variables for African American and Latin American, with European American omitted. Parents' highest level of education was computed from both mother and father data into three values: (1) at least one parent had more than a high school education, (2) at least one parent had a high school education or GED, (3) both parents had less than a high school education. Additional covariates (above the federal poverty level at baseline, mother is other race, either parent was a teenager at child's birth, and parents' biological status) were entered in initial analyses but omitted due to nonsignificance.

Analytic Plan

Intercorrelations among parenting scales were computed separately for mothers and fathers to examine patterns of covariation at the bivariate level. We then used K-means cluster analysis to identify naturally occurring patterns in parenting style at the multivariate level among all six parenting scales, again separately for mothers and fathers. The K-means method was preferable to a hierarchical method because of the relatively large sample size (Aldenderfer & Blashfield, 1984; Jain & Dubes, 1988). Solutions with two, three, and four groups were attempted. The solution that allowed for the most distinct, theoretically meaningful cluster groups to emerge was ultimately selected.

Once the optimal clustering solutions for mothers and fathers were identified, ANCOVAs were used to compute adjusted means of children's

MDI scores by mother and father parenting cluster separately. Mother race, highest parent education, child gender, and program status were held constant at their means in all analyses. Next, mother and father clusters were cross-classified within couples to create mother – father parenting pairs. To examine whether child outcomes varied according to particular combinations of mother and father parenting style, ANCOVAs were used to compute adjusted means for child outcomes by mother and father cluster pair.

RESULTS

Cluster Analysis of Parenting Scales

The intercorrelations among parenting scales were remarkably similar for mothers and fathers overall (not shown).[3] Cognitive stimulation was moderately correlated with positive regard for both parents, but its correlation with sensitivity was stronger for mothers than fathers, *rs* = .71 versus .58, $z = 2.43$, $p < .05$. Moreover, the negative correlations between cognitive stimulation and intrusiveness, detachment, and negative regard were stronger for mothers than fathers. Therefore, cognitive stimulation had a stronger linear relation to positive behaviors and a weaker relation to negative ones for mothers than for fathers. In addition, the correlation between intrusiveness and negative regard was stronger among fathers than mothers, *rs* = .51 versus .36, $z = 2.01$, $p < .05$. It may be that intrusiveness is driven more by an impulse to teach than it is by feelings of hostility among mothers.

Consistent with the correlation analysis of the six parenting scales by gender, the cluster analyses run separately for mothers and fathers produced similar parenting patterns. Four clusters emerged within each gender (Table 1). For both genders, there was a group we termed *Highly Supportive* that had the highest mean scores on the positive scales (sensitivity, cognitive stimulation, and positive regard) and the lowest mean scores on the negative ones (intrusiveness, negative regard, and detachment). A group also emerged within each gender that we termed *Somewhat Supportive,* which scored second highest on the positive scales and second lowest on the negative ones. It should be noted that the clusters were distinguished from each other not only by their relative mean scores on the parenting scales across clusters, but also by the scores of the scales relative to each other within each cluster. That is, clusters differed according to

---

[3]A table of intercorrelations among parenting scales for mothers and fathers is available from first author on request.

TABLE 1
Parenting Scale Score by Cluster

	Mothers						Fathers					
	Full	Highly Supportive (*n* = 101)	Somewhat Supportive (*n* = 82)	Negative (*n* = 34)	Detached (*n* = 20)	*F*	Full	Highly Supportive (*n* = 80)	Somewhat Supportive (*n* = 102)	Negative (*n* = 19)	Detached (*n* = 36)	*F*
Sensitivity	4.9	5.7	4.7	3.8	3.3	140.3	4.6	5.5	4.6	3.2	3.4	142.3
	(1.0)	(0.6)	(0.6)	(0.8)	(0.7)		(1.0)	(0.6)	(0.6)	(0.7)	(0.7)	
Positive regard	3.9	5.0	3.4	2.9	2.2	134.6	3.6	5.0	3.3	2.4	1.9	193.1
	(1.3)	(0.8)	(0.7)	(0.9)	(0.7)		(1.4)	(0.8)	(0.7)	(0.7)	(0.5)	
Cognitive stimulation	4.2	5.0	3.9	3.6	2.3	96.5	4.0	4.8	3.9	3.5	2.8	66.9
	(1.1)	(0.7)	(0.7)	(0.8)	(0.6)		(1.0)	(0.8)	(0.7)	(0.8)	(0.5)	
Negative regard	1.3	1.1	1.3	1.9	1.7	17.7	1.3	1.1	1.2	2.5	1.3	49.2
	(0.7)	(0.3)	(0.6)	(0.9)	(1.2)		(0.6)	(0.3)	(0.4)	(0.9)	(0.6)	
Intrusiveness	1.8	1.4	1.5	3.5	1.4	106.3	1.8	1.5	1.8	4.0	1.6	61.8
	(0.9)	(0.6)	(0.6)	(0.8)	(0.7)		(1.0)	(0.6)	(0.7)	(0.9)	(0.8)	
Detachment	1.3	1.1	1.2	1.3	2.9	89.0	1.2	1.0	1.2	1.4	1.9	26.7
	(0.7)	(0.2)	(0.5)	(0.5)	(1.0)		(0.6)	(0.2)	(0.4)	(0.8)	(0.9)	

Note. Standard deviations are displayed in parentheses below means for each parenting cluster; all *F*s are significant at $p < .001$.

the shape of scores across scales as well as the height of individual scale scores. For example, among both mothers and fathers, the Highly Supportive and Somewhat Supportive clusters scored higher than other clusters on the positive scales; in addition, within these two clusters, all positive scale scores were higher than negative scale scores.

By contrast, two clusters emerged among both mothers and fathers for whom a negative scale score was high relative to the positive scale scores. Among mothers and fathers, these groups were termed *Negative* and *Detached.* The Negative mother cluster scored far higher than the other three mother clusters on both negative regard and intrusiveness. Similarly, the Negative father cluster scored highest on those two scales among fathers. However, Negative mothers were slightly more sensitive than they were intrusive, and were equally cognitively stimulating. By contrast, Negative fathers were far more intrusive than they were stimulating or sensitive. That is, the Negative father group was characterized foremost by intrusiveness. Among mothers, the Detached cluster scored far higher than the other clusters on detachment. In addition, after sensitivity, detachment was their next highest scoring scale. Among fathers, the Detached cluster scored higher than the other clusters on detachment. However, within the Detached cluster, detachment was tied for third place after sensitivity and cognitive stimulation as the highest scoring scale.

Although the clusters for mothers and fathers resembled each other, it is not the case that mothers and fathers scored similarly overall on parenting scales. For example, both genders yielded a Highly Supportive cluster, but that cluster was the largest among women (n = 101, 43%) and the second largest (n = 80, 34%) among men. The plurality of men were Somewhat Supportive (n = 102, 43%), whereas among women that group was second largest (n = 82, 35%). The fewest mothers were Detached (n = 20, 8%), and the fewest fathers were Negative (n = 19, 8%).

Child Outcomes by Cluster

Children's cognitive scores at 24 and 36 months are presented in Table 2, first according to their mother's cluster, and then according to their father's. Both unadjusted and adjusted means are presented. Differences emerged across mother clusters as early as 24 months, with a spread of 9.1 points on the adjusted MDI between the highest (Highly Supportive) and lowest (Detached) scoring clusters ($p < .05$). Children of Highly Supportive mothers scored highest, those of Somewhat Supportive mothers scored next highest, and those of Detached and Negative mothers scored lowest. By 36 months, the spread on the adjusted MDI grew to 12.2 points ($p < .05$). Children of Highly Supportive mothers continued to score highest,

TABLE 2
Child Outcomes at 24 and 36 Months by Mother and Father Parenting Cluster

	24 Months Bayley MDI				36 Months Bayley MDI			
	M[a]	*F*	*M* (Adj)[b]	*F*	*M*[a]	*F*	*M* (Adj)[b]	*F*
Mothers		8.8***		3.9**		10.6***		5.9***
Highly Supportive	96.7_1		95.2_1		98.9_1		97.5_1	
	(13.6)		(1.4)		(13.3)		(1.4)	
Somewhat Supportive	$91.5_{1,2}$		$92.1_{1,2}$		90.4_2		90.8_2	
	(13.5)		(1.6)		(12.6)		(1.5)	
Negative	83.1_2		86.5_2		87.5_2		90.4_2	
	(14.9)		(2.7)		(12.5)		(2.3)	
Detached	85.2_2		86.1_2		84.7_2		85.3_2	
	(15.1)		(3.4)		(11.9)		(3.3)	
Fathers		5.2**		2.0		8.1***		5.3**
Highly Supportive	96.5_1		95.1		98.6_1		97.2_1	
	(15.1)		(1.6)		(13.7)		(1.5)	
Somewhat Supportive	$91.9_{1,2}$		91.9		92.3_2		$92.3_{1,2}$	
	(13.4)		(1.5)		(12.0)		(1.4)	
Negative	84.1_2		88.2		88.8_2		$93.0_{1,2}$	
	(13.7)		(3.4)		(10.5)		(3.2)	
Detached	87.9_2		89.2		85.7_2		86.6_2	
	(14.3)		(2.4)		(15.3)		(2.2)	

Note. $N = 212$ for 24-month Bayley MDI; $N = 196$ for 36-month Bayley MDI; for each outcome, different subscripts across clusters denote significant differences at $p < .10$ in post-hoc Bonferroni-adjusted pairwise comparisons.

[a]Means are unadjusted; standard deviations are displayed below means in parentheses.

[b]Means are adjusted for child sex, maternal race, highest parental education and program status; standard errors are displayed below means in parentheses.

**$p < .01$. ***$p < .001$.

whereas those of Detached mothers scored lowest of all. Children of Somewhat Supportive and Negative mothers scored similarly. A similar pattern emerged according to father cluster. At 24 months, the spread on the adjusted MDI between the highest (Highly Supportive) and lowest (Negative) was 6.9 points, although this difference was not statistically significant. By 36 months, it had grown to 10.6 points ($p < .05$). As with mothers, children of Highly Supportive fathers scored highest, those of Detached fathers scored lowest, and those of Somewhat Supportive and Negative fathers scored similarly.

Child Outcomes by Cluster Pairs

To this point, all analyses treated mother and father clusters separately. At this stage, mother – father pairs were created by cross-classifying each partner's cluster membership. Because there were four mother and four father clusters, cross-classification resulted in 16 combinations, several with prohibitively small cells ($n < 5$). To enable the meaningful comparison of children's cognitive scores according to their mother – father combination, we aggregated cells to the greatest extent possible. First, among both mothers and fathers, the Highly Supportive and Somewhat Supportive clusters were merged into a single Supportive cluster because they scored similarly on parenting scales relative to the other clusters, suggesting that they represented points on a continuum rather than discrete categories. To test the effect of a single Supportive parent, children with a Supportive mother whose father was Detached or Negative were aggregated into a single group. Similarly, children with a Supportive father and a Detached or Negative mother were consolidated. Finally, children with no Supportive parents (i.e., with two Negative or Detached parents) were consolidated.

These consolidations resulted in a total of four mother – father combinations: (1) Supportive mother and Supportive father ($n = 147$, 62%), (2) Supportive mother and Unsupportive father ($n = 36$, 15%), (3) Supportive father and Unsupportive mother ($n = 35$, 15%), and (4) Two Unsupportive parents ($n = 19$, 8%).

Figures 1 and 2 present children's mean MDI scores at 24 and 36 months for these four groups, adjusted for maternal race, highest parental education, child sex, and program status. All ANCOVAs were also run excluding highest parent education as a covariate; it was hypothesized that parent education level influences parenting style to an extent that controlling for it may obscure important differences among parenting clusters and variations in child outcomes as a result. However, results of analyses excluding parent education did not substantively alter our conclusions. Analyses show that children of two Supportive parents consistently scored the high-

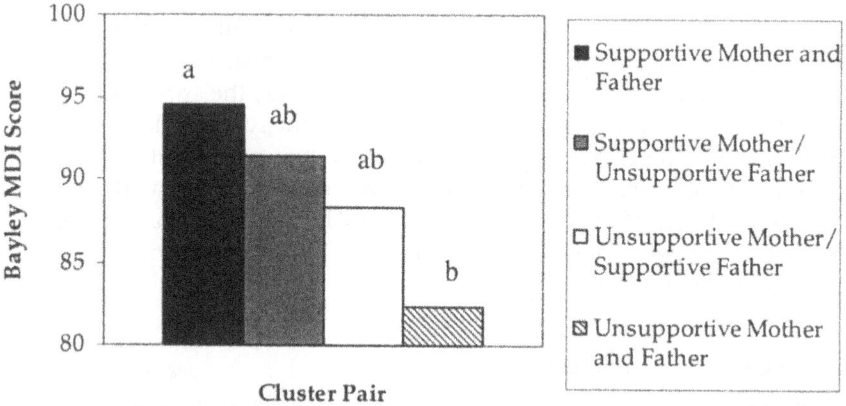

FIGURE 1

Mean 24-month Bayley Mental Development Index score by parenting cluster pair. Different letters indicate significant differences at $p < .05$ in post hoc Bonferroni-adjusted pairwise comparisons.

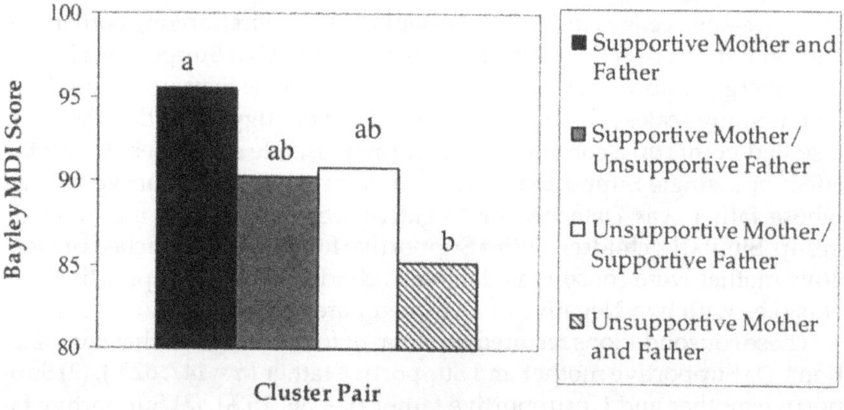

FIGURE 2

Mean 36-month Bayley Mental Development Index score by parenting cluster pair. Different letters indicate significant differences at $p < .05$ in post hoc Bonferroni-adjusted pairwise comparisons.

est, and children of two Unsupportive parents consistently scored the lowest on cognitive tests in early childhood. The difference between them remained relatively consistent over time (12.2 points at 24 months, $p < .05$, and 10.4 points at 36 months, $p < .05$). Additionally, program status was a significant covariate in all ANCOVAs for 36-month MDI scores; children in the program group scored higher than those in the control group ($p < .05$).

Children of two Supportive parents also had higher cognitive test scores than those with either a Supportive mother or Supportive father only, although not with statistical significance. On the 36-month MDI, for example, children of two Supportive parents scored $M = 95.5$, compared to children with a Supportive father only, $M = 90.8$, or mother only, $M = 90.2$. Although these contrasts were not statistically significant, the consistency of the advantage suggests a particular benefit for children with two Supportive parents.

Among children with one Supportive parent, there was no clear advantage according to the Supportive parent's gender. Although children with a Supportive mother scored slightly higher than those with a Supportive father on the 24-month MDI, these differences were slight and not statistically significant, and they did not appear at 36 months. Both groups scored higher than those with no Supportive parents at 24 and 36 months, although these differences were not statistically significant.

To assess more directly the advantages associated with number of Supportive parents, children with a Supportive mother and father ($n = 147$) were compared to those with only one Supportive parent (mother or father; $n = 71$) as well as those with none ($n = 19$). At 24 months, children with two Supportive parents scored 4.6 points higher than those with only one Supportive parent ($p = .10$) and 12.2 points higher than those with no Supportive parents ($p < .01$), after controlling for maternal race, highest parental education, child gender, and program status (not shown). Children with one Supportive parent scored 7.6 points higher than those with none, although this difference was not statistically significant. At 36 months, children with two Supportive parents scored 5 points higher than both those with one Supportive parent ($p < .05$) and 10.4 points higher than those with none ($p < .05$). At this time point, children with only one Supportive parent scored 5.4 points higher than children with no Supportive parents, although, as at 24 months, this difference did not reach statistical significance.

DISCUSSION

This study examined parenting patterns in a sample of low-income couples and the impact of those patterns on young children's cognitive outcomes. Cluster analyses revealed that overall patterns of parenting were similar among mothers and fathers. However, the profiles of the Detached and Negative clusters differed by gender. Negative fathers were more intrusive than Negative mothers, and Detached fathers were less detached than Detached mothers. Additionally, the plurality of mothers fell into the

Highly Supportive cluster, whereas an almost equal proportion of fathers fell into the Somewhat Supportive one.

Child cognitive outcomes were associated with the four clusters similarly among mothers and fathers. Specifically, the children of Highly Supportive mothers scored highest at 24 and 36 months, as did the children of Highly Supportive fathers. By 36 months, the children of Detached mothers scored lowest, as did the children of Detached fathers. Interscale correlations (not shown) revealed that, among both mothers and fathers, detachment was more negatively correlated with cognitive stimulation than was intrusiveness or negative regard. This may account for the relative disadvantage of Detached parents' children compared to Negative parents' children. For this reason, however, this finding may be specific to cognitive outcomes; perhaps the provision of cognitive stimulation is less important for other types of outcomes, such as socioemotional ones.

The associations between parenting style and child outcomes that were obtained with each parent separately are even stronger when mother and father parenting are considered together. First, the advantage of having a Supportive parent is compounded by the presence of another Supportive parent. At both time points, children of two Supportive parents scored higher than children with only one (significantly so only at 36 months and only when the Supportive-mother-only and Supportive-father-only groups were combined), suggesting a genuine advantage conferred by two Supportive parents compared to one. A second Supportive parent may augment the benefits of the first because he or she establishes a consistently positive parenting milieu without Negative or Detached interactions for the child to negotiate. Alternatively, Supportive parent pairs may have superior interpersonal skills and emotional well-being, and thus enjoy higher quality relationships; better parental relationship quality, in turn, is associated with more positive child outcomes (Belsky, 1984; Cummings & Davies, 1994).

Second, we find that among children with only one Supportive parent, it appears not to matter whether that parent is the mother or father. This result is surprising in light of the conventional wisdom that considers mother behavior more influential than father behavior for child development. Our results should be interpreted in light of the composition of this sample, which is extremely selective of highly involved fathers. It may be that for a population with greater variability in father involvement, the benefits of having only a Supportive mother outweigh those of having only a Supportive father.

Third, we find that children with one Supportive parent scored consistently higher than those with none, suggesting that the disadvantage of having an Unsupportive parent is compounded by having a second

Unsupportive parent. Although, this contrast never reached statistical significance, the difference in scores between children with one Supportive parent and none was greater than or equal to the difference between those with two Supportive parents and one at both time points.

A limitation of this study was the consolidation of clusters mandated by small cell sizes in the analysis of mother – father pairs. For example, Highly Supportive and Somewhat Supportive parents were combined into a single Supportive group. In separate mother and father cluster analyses, however, children with Somewhat Supportive parents scored lower than children with Highly Supportive parents and similarly to those with Negative parents. Therefore, differences between children with two versus one Supportive parent may be larger than these analyses suggest. Future research with a larger sample is needed to distinguish the effects of Highly Supportive parents from those of Somewhat Supportive ones.

Despite the selective nature of the sample, these findings are relevant to a discussion of low-income families with two involved parents. Such families are often the targets, and most engaged consumers, of intervention services like Early Head Start. Our findings regarding the benefit of two Supportive parents suggest that attempts to improve parenting skills should include fathers as well as mothers, and that practitioners should address both parents' behaviors in concert.

AFFILIATIONS AND ADDRESSES

Rebecca M. Ryan, Teachers College, Columbia University, 525 West 120th Street, Box 39, New York, NY 10027. E-mail: Rmr133@columbia.edu. Anne Martin and Jeanne Brooks-Gunn are also at Columbia University.

ACKNOWLEDGMENTS

The findings reported here are based on research conducted as part of the national Early Head Start Research and Evaluation Project funded by the Administration for Children and Families (ACF), U.S. Department of Health and Human Services under contract 105–95–1936 to Mathematica Policy Research, Princeton, NJ, and Columbia University's National Center for Children and Families, Teachers College, in conjunction with the Early Head Start Research Consortium. The Consortium consists of representatives from 17 programs participating in the evaluation, 15 local research teams, the evaluation contractors, and ACF. Research institutions in the Consortium (and principal researchers for conducting the research through 36 months of age) include ACF (Rachel Chazan Cohen, Judith Jerald, Esther Kresh, Helen Raikes, and Louisa Tarullo); Catholic University of America (Michaela Farber, Harriet Liebow, Nancy Taylor, Elizabeth Timberlake, and Shavaun Wall); Columbia University (Lisa Berlin, Christy Brady-Smith, Jeanne Brooks-Gunn, and Allison Sidle Fuligni); Harvard University (Catherine Ayoub, Barbara Alexander Pan, and Catherine Snow); Iowa State University (Dee Draper, Gayle Luze, Susan McBride, and Carla Peterson); Mathematica Policy Research (Kimberly Boller, Jill Constantine, Ellen Eliason Kisker, John M. Love, Diane Paulsell, Christine Ross, Peter Schochet, Cheri Vogel, and Welmoet van Kammen); Medical University of South Carolina (Richard Faldowski, Gui-Young Hong, and Susan Pickrel); Michigan State University (Hiram Fitzgerald, Tom Reischl, and Rachel Schiffman); New York University (Mark Spellmann and Catherine Tamis-LeMonda); University of Arkansas (Robert Bradley, Richard Clubb, Andrea Hart, Mark Swanson, and Leanne Whiteside-Mansell); University of California, Los Angeles (Carollee Howes and Claire Hamilton); University of Colorado Health Sciences Center (Robert Emde, Jon Korfmacher, JoAnn Robinson, Paul Spicer, and Norman Watt); University of Kansas (Jane Atwater, Judith Carta, and Jean Ann Summers); University of Missouri–Columbia (Mark Fine, Jean Ispa, and Kathy Thornburg); University of Pittsburgh (Beth Green, Carol McAllister, and Robert McCall); University of Washington School of Education (Eduardo Armijo and Joseph Stowitschek); University of Washington School of Nursing (Kathryn Barnard and Susan Spieker); and Utah State University (Lisa Boyce, Gina Cook, Catherine Callow-Heusser, and Lori Roggman).

The authors thank the Consortium members who reviewed and commented on an earlier draft of this article, as well as members of the Early Head Start Consortium Father Working Group. The content of this publication does not necessarily reflect the views or policies of the Department of Health and Human Services, and mention of trade names, commercial products, or organizations does not imply endorsement by the U.S. Government.

REFERENCES

Aldenderfer, M. S., & Blashfield, R. K. (1984). *Cluster analysis.* Newbury Park, CA: Sage.

Ban, P. L., & Lewis, M. (1974). Mothers and fathers, girls and boys: Attachment behavior in the one-year-old. *Merrill-Palmer Quarterly, 20,* 195–204.

Belsky, J. (1979). Mother–father–infant interaction: A naturalistic observation study. *Developmental Psychology, 15,* 601–607.

Belsky, J. (1984). The determinants of parenting: A process model. *Child Development, 55,* 83–96.

Belsky, J., Gilstrap, B., & Rovine, M. (1984). The Pennsylvania Infant and Family Development Project, I: Stability and change in mother–infant and father–infant interaction in a family setting at one, three, and nine months. *Child Development, 55,* 692–705.

Bentley, K. S., & Fox, R. A. (1991). Mothers and fathers of young children: Comparison of parenting styles. *Psychological Reports, 69,* 320–322.

Black, M. M., Dubowitz, H., & Starr, R. H. (1999). African American fathers in low income, urban families: Development, behavior, and home environment of their three-year-old children. *Child Development, 70,* 967–978.

Bornstein, M. (Ed.). (2002). *Handbook of parenting, Vol. 1: Children and parenting* (2nd ed., pp. 3–43). Mahwah, NJ: Lawrence Erlbaum Associates, Inc.

Brady-Smith, C., O-Brien, C., Berlin, L., & Ware, A. (1999). *24-Month Child–Parent Interaction Rating Scales for the Three-Bag Assessment.* New York: Teachers College Press.

Cabrera, N., Brooks-Gunn, J., Moore, K., West, J., Boller, K., & Tamis-LeMonda, C. (2002). Bridging research and policy: Including fathers of young children in national studies. In C. Tamis-LeMonda & N. Cabrera (Eds.), *Handbook of father involvement: Multidisciplinary perspectives* (pp. 5–3). Mahwah, NJ: Lawrence Erlbaum Associates, Inc.

Conner, D. B., Knight, D. K., & Cross, D. R. (1997). Mothers' and fathers' scaffolding of their 2-year-olds during problem-solving and literacy interactions. *British Journal of Developmental Psychology, 15,* 323–338.

Cummings, E. M., & Davies, P. (1994). *Children and marital conflict: The impact of dispute and resolution.* New York: Guilford.

Darling, N., & Steinberg, L. (1993). Parenting style as context: An integrative model. *Psychological Bulletin, 113*(3), 487–496.

De Wolff, M. S., & van Ijzendoorn, M. H. (1997). Sensitivity and attachment: A meta-analysis on parental antecedents of infant attachment. *Child Development, 68,* 571–591.

Duncan, G. J., & Brooks-Gunn, J. (Eds.). (1997). *Consequences of growing up poor.* New York: Russell Sage Foundation.

Elder, G. H., Jr. (1974). *Children of the great depression: Social change in life experience.* Chicago: University of Chicago Press.

Jain, A. K., & Dubes, R. C. (1988). *Algorithms for clustering data.* Englewood Cliffs, NJ: Prentice Hall.

Kelley, M. L., Smith, T. S., Green, A. P., Berndt, A. E., & Rogers, M. C. (1998). Importance of fathers' parenting to African–American toddler's social and cognitive development. *Infant Behavior and Development, 21,* 733–744.

Lamb, M. (1997). Infant–father attachments and their impact on child development. In M. Lamb (Ed.), *The role of the father in child development* (3rd ed., pp. 93–117). New York: Wiley.

Lamb, M., Frodi, A.M., Hwang, C., Frodi, M., & Steinberg, J. (1982). Mother- and father–infant interaction involving play and holding in traditional and nontraditional Swedish families. *Developmental Psychology, 18,* 215–221.

Landry, S. H., Smith, K. E., Swank, P. R., Assel, M. A., & Vellet, S. (2001). Does early responsive parenting have a special importance for children's development or is consistency across early childhood necessary? *Developmental Psychology, 37,* 387–403.

National Institute of Child Health and Human Development Early Child Care Research Network. (1999). Chronicity of maternal depressive symptoms, maternal sensitivity, and child functioning at 36 months. *Developmental Psychology, 35,* 1297–1310.

Padilla, Y., & Reichman, N. (2001). Low birthweight: Do unwed fathers help? *Children and Youth Services Review, 23,* 427–452.

Pettit, G. S., Bates, J. E., & Dodge, K. A. (1997). Supportive parenting, ecological context, and children's adjustment: A seven-year longitudinal study. *Child Development, 68,* 908–923.

Power, T. G., & Parke, R. D. (1983). Patterns of mother and father play with their 8-month-old infant: A multiple analyses approach. *Infant Behavior and Development, 8,* 453–459.

Rothbaum, F., & Weisz, J. (1994). Parental converging and child externalizing behavior in non-clinical samples: A meta-analysis. *Psychological Bulletin, 116,* 55–74.

Shannon, J. D., Tamis-LeMonda, C. S., London, K., & Cabrera, N. (2002). Beyond rough and tumble: Low-income fathers' interactions and children's cognitive development at 24 months. *Parenting: Science and Practice, 2,* 77–104.

Tamis-LeMonda, C., Shannon, J. D., Cabrera, N., & Lamb, M. (2004). Fathers and mothers at play with their 2-year-olds: Contributions to language and cognitive development. *Child Development, 75,* 1806–1820.

Vandell, D. L. (1979). A microanalysis of toddlers' social interaction with mothers and fathers. *Journal of Genetic Psychology, 134*(2), 299–312.

Ventura, S. J., & Bachrach, C. A. (2000). Nonmarital childbearing in the United States, 1940–1999. *National Vital Statistics Reports, 48,* 16. Washington, DC: National Center for Health Statistics.

Yogman, M., Kindlon, D., & Earls, F. (1995). Father involvement and cognitive/behavioral outcomes of preterm infants. *Journal of the American Academy of Child & Adolescent Psychiatry, 34,* 58–66.

PARENTING: SCIENCE AND PRACTICE
April–September 2006 Volume 6 Number 2 & 3 Pages 229–242

Two Studies of Father Involvement in Early Head Start Programs: A National Survey and a Demonstration Program Evaluation

Helen H. Raikes and Jeanne Bellotti

SYNOPSIS

Objective. Departing from the typical focus of intervention studies on service use and program effects for mothers and children, this article examines the extent to which fathers are present as clients in Early Head Start intervention programs for infants and toddlers. ***Design.*** The article uses descriptive findings from 2 studies: the first is a population survey of 261 Early Head Start programs (National Practitioners Survey), and the second is a father involvement demonstration program of 21 programs (Fatherhood Demonstration Study). Similar measures enabled comparability across the studies. ***Results.*** The 2 studies report that there was a father present in the lives of a majority of Early Head Start children — 70% in the national study, and 76% in the demonstration study. However, only 45% and 48%, respectively, of children had a father in residence, and there was considerable variation by race and ethnicity. About 59% of resident fathers had some participation in programs (53% in demonstration programs). Demonstration programs involved more nonresident fathers (45%) than did typical programs (30%). The proportion of resident fathers who were involved in Early Head Start at higher levels, defined in this study as at least 3 times a month, equaled 24% and 48% for typical and demonstration programs, respectively. For nonresident fathers, comparable figures were 10% and 30%. ***Conclusions.*** These studies illustrate that the majority of Early Head Start children have a father present in their lives, although many fathers are not in residence, and that the majority of fathers have some contact with the program. Findings showing that demonstration programs were more successful in engaging fathers at higher levels of involvement (especially true for nonresident fathers) illustrate that there is a greater potential for father participation in intervention programs than is realized today. Greater inclusion of fathers as clients in these programs has important implications for the science and practice of intervention.

INTRODUCTION

The science of early intervention has demonstrated that it is possible to enhance parenting and children's development through intensive and comprehensive intervention programs (Administration for Children and Families [ACF], 2002a; Kitzman et al., 2000; Ramey & Campbell, 1991). Surprisingly, this science is built almost exclusively on what is known about intervening with mothers and children. Only recently has the focus expanded to include fathers (Fagan & Iglesias, 1999; Fagan & Palm, 2004; Mahoney, Wiggers, & Lash, 1996), important given the contributions of fathers to the development of low-income children (Black, Dubowitz, & Starr, 1999; Tamis-LeMonda, Shannon, Cabrera, & Lamb, 2004). Here we examine data drawn from all Early Head Start sites to address the extent of father presence in the lives of Early Head Start children and their level of involvement in Early Head Start programs. We conducted our investigation in the wider population of Early Head Start (as of 2004, over 700 programs), because of the low incidence of many father involvement activities found in research sites (Cohen & Love, 1999). A larger sample also enables study of variations in father characteristics and program involvement. The first set of findings presented in this article are from a national survey of father involvement in Early Head Start programs (Raikes, Boller, van Kammen, & Summers, 2002), the National Practitioners Survey. The findings provide a population baseline for our second study, the Fatherhood Demonstration Study of programs receiving additional resources and training for father involvement.

In 2001, the Head Start Bureau along with the Office of Child Support Enforcement funded 21 Fatherhood Demonstration sites with special resources for father involvement in the Early Head Start program. The evaluation of the Fatherhood Demonstration sites was conducted by Mathematica Policy Research and utilized the survey instrument from the National Practitioners Study (Bellotti et al., 2003).

This article addresses the same questions across two studies using similar methods: (1) To what extent are fathers present in the lives of Early Head Start children? Does involvement vary by racial and cultural characteristics? (2) To what extent do fathers participate in Early Head Start programs? What kinds of services do they use? What are average levels of father involvement in programs?

STUDY 1

Sample and Procedures

In the winter of 1999 to 2000, all Early Head Start programs serving children and families were invited to complete a survey about fathers of Early

Head Start children and father program participation. Of 416 eligible programs at that time, 261 completed the survey, for a 63% response rate. Noncompleters tended to be recently funded programs not yet offering full services or those not offering father involvement activities.

The sample of sites participating in the study was diverse and included those funded from 1995 to 1999: 26% were center-based, 37% home-based, and 37% were mixed-approach programs (in which some families received center-based services and some home-based or both). The programs served diverse racial groups: 23% served predominantly African American families, 13% Latin American families, 44% European American, 4% Native American, and 15% of the programs served a mixture of racial groups (defined as having no group represented at greater than 50%). The programs in this sample were more often serving families in rural areas or small towns (71%) versus urban areas. In 17% of the programs, between one quarter and one half of the parents were teens, and in 11% of the programs, more than one half of the parents were teens. The programs served 75 children, on average (see Table 1). These characteristics of Early Head Start programs are typical of all programs that were providing services at the time (ACF, 2002b; ACYF, 1999, 2000).

Data from other Early Head Start research had shown that programs pass through distinguishable stages in father involvement (McAllister, Wilson, & Burton, 2004). Therefore, we asked program directors to classify their programs using the following scale:

(1) Prestage: Little thought given to the unique issues of involving any parent beyond the mother.

(2) Early: Some fathers involved, but most program activities still revolve around women and children.

(3) Midstage: Program has begun to show a concerted effort to involve fathers. Some changes are occurring as more staff and parents gain a sense of how to make the program father-friendly. Father Involvement Coordinator may be hired and does a good job of keeping other staff aware of father involvement.

(4) Mature: Many changes have been made in making the program father-friendly. Father involvement now focuses on applying all program activities to fathers. Many resident fathers are now involved with the program. Some nonresident fathers are involved.

(5) Very Mature: Most resident fathers are involved in the program on at least a monthly basis. The program offers a great variety of father-involvement activities. Many nonresident fathers are involved.

Seventy-two percent of the programs classified themselves as "Prestage" or "Early" in development of father program involvement, 21% were clas-

TABLE 1
Program, Child, and Father Characteristics

	National Practitioners Survey		Fatherhood Demonstration Study
	Total	Mature Programs	Total[a]
Program approach			
Home-based	36.8	29.4	31.6
Center-based	25.7	17.6	52.6
Mixed	37.5	52.9	15.8
Service delivery area			
Rural	70.5	55.5	26.3
Urban	29.5	44.4	73.7
Race or ethnicity of enrolled children			
African American	22.7	44.4	34.3
Latin American	12.6	11.1	38.4
European American	44.3	11.1	16.4
Native American	4.3	11.1	5.5
Mixture of racial groups	15.3	22.2	5.5
Proportion of teen parents			
25% or fewer	71.5	44.4	63.1
26% to 50%	17.4	27.8	31.6
51% to 100%	11.1	27.8	5.3
Number of children served	75.4	105.1	105.1
Sample size (programs)	261	18	19

Note. Percentage of Programs unless otherwise indicated. This information was provided by the Early Head Start National Practitioners Survey and the Evaluation of the Early Head Start Fatherhood Demonstration.

[a]Data reflect the responses of Early Head Start directors or designates. Nineteen of the 21 Early Head Start directors completed the survey as part of the Evaluation of the Fatherhood Demonstration.

sified as "Midstage," and 7% were "Mature or Very Mature." We report findings for all the programs in the study and for "Mature" and "Very Mature" programs (referred to as mature programs). Programs that were mature in father friendliness were slightly larger than typical programs (serving 104 children on average), more often early funded programs, mixed-approach, primarily serving African American families, and somewhat more likely to be in urban areas than less mature programs.

Results

Programs reported that the majority of children had a father or father figure involved in their lives (70%). About 45% of children in the sample had a resident father, whereas 25% were reported to have a nonresident but involved father (defined as seeing or communicating with the child several times over the past 3 months). These percentages were similar to rates reported in the 17-site Early Head Start sample by mother report (Cabrera et al., 2004). We found considerable variation across Early Head Start programs in the proportion of children with a resident father. In programs serving predominantly African American families, 30% of children were reported to have a resident father (37% reported involved, nonresident fathers). Programs serving predominantly Latin American families reported 57% of children with a resident father (24% reported involved, nonresident fathers). Programs serving mostly European American families had 48% resident fathers (20% had involved, nonresident fathers). The lowest proportion of children with involved fathers were in Native American programs—47% resident and 16% involved, nonresident fathers. The programs serving mixed racial groups were similar to those serving European Americans and Latin Americans, with 46% resident fathers (26% involved, nonresident). Programs serving families in rural areas reported greater involvement of resident fathers in children's lives than was true for programs in urban areas, 47% versus 39%. Slightly more than one third of the programs (37%) served some fathers who were primary caregivers of their children. Most reported only one or two of these custodial fathers, but 18 programs reported three or more. Programs that classified themselves as mature in terms of father involvement activities were no different from other programs in the percentage of children who had resident fathers, or in the number or likelihood of serving children with custodial fathers.

Next, we inquired about the extent of father participation in the program. As seen in Table 2, 59% of resident fathers were reported to have had ever participated in the Early Head Start program. Of nonresident fathers, 30% had some participation. Nearly a quarter (24%) of the fathers had high levels of participation (attended three or more events a month). Even 10% of nonresident fathers had high levels of participation in program activities. When asked to account for specific ways fathers participated, mature programs substantiated that more resident fathers participated (65%), participated at high levels (41%), and more nonresident fathers participated at high levels (14%) than was true for the programs in earlier stages of father involvement. However, nonresident fathers were no more likely to ever participate in mature than in other programs.

To explore participation patterns in more detail, we asked programs to identify the extent to which fathers participated in specific types of activities, and scores were summed to create two scales as described earlier. The average score on the Father Program Activities Scale of all 23 father involvement items was 1.6, indicating that few fathers were involved in typical activities queried (Table 3). Scores for mature programs were signifi-

TABLE 2
Father Involvement With Their Children and Early Head Start
(Percentage of Programs)

	National Practitioners Survey		Fatherhood Demonstration Study
	Total	Mature Programs	Total[a]
Percentage of programs that try to involve			
Resident biological	98.8	100.0	100.0
Resident father figures	94.8	100.0	100.0
Nonresident biological	77.2	88.9	94.7
Nonresident father figures	57.9	83.3	84.2
Percentage of programs that make a strong effort to involve incarcerated fathers	10.1	40.0	26.3
Resident fathers and father figures			
Percentage of children with a resident father or father figure	44.6 (22.4)	36.2 (20.0)	47.1 (21.1)
Percentage of children with resident father or father figure who ever participated in Early Head Start[b]	58.6 (28.8)	65.4 (25.4)	53.2 (26.0)
Percentage of children with a highly involved resident father or father figure[b]	24.1 (21.1)	41.2 (32.4)	48.3 (31.3)
Nonresident fathers and father figures			
Percentage of children with an involved, nonresident father or father figure	24.9 (20.2)	41.0 (28.6)	28.8 (22.0)
Percentage of children with an involved, nonresident father or father figure who ever participated in Early Head Start[c]	30.4 (29.8)	26.6 (23.0)	45.3 (26.8)
Percentage of children with a highly involved, nonresident father or father figure[c]	9.5 (17.8)	13.5 (17.4)	29.6 (32.3)
Percentage of children living in a father-only household	1.2 (3.1)	0.7 (1.2)	0.9 (1.3)
Sample size (Programs)	261	18	19

Note. Early Head Start National Practitioners Survey and the Evaluation of the Early Head Start Fatherhood Demonstration Study.

[a]Data reflect the responses of Early Head Start directors or designates. Nineteen of the 21 Early Head Start directors completed the survey as part of the Evaluation of the Fatherhood Demonstration.

[b]Data pertain to only those children who have a resident father or father figure. Highly involved in the Early Head Start program was defined as participation three or more times a month in different program activities.

[c]Data pertain to only those children who have an involved, nonresident father. Involved, nonresident father or father figure was defined as seeing or communicating with the child a few times a month over the past 3 months.

TABLE 3

Father Participation in Early Head Start Activities (Average Scale Scores[a])

	National Practitioners Survey				Fatherhood Demonstration Study	
	Total		Mature Programs		Total[b]	
	M	*SD*	*M*	*SD*	*M*	*SD*
Father program activities scale	1.61	0.5	2.10	.4	2.26	0.4
Father-focused program activities scale score	0.62	0.9	2.04	.9	2.37	0.4
Father participation in specific activities						
Applying for the program	2.01	0.7	2.39	0.8	2.00	0.8
Family activities	2.72	1.0	3.56	0.7	3.04	0.8
Activities to improve parenting	2.06	0.9	3.17	0.7	2.62	0.7
Group parenting education	2.30	1.0	3.17	0.9	2.67	0.9
Activities for fathers and children[c]	0.82	1.3	2.56	1.7	2.50	1.2
Sporting events[c]	0.56	1.1	1.72	1.5	2.26	1.6
Men's group focused on parenting[c]	0.70	1.1	2.44	1.4	2.61	1.0
Men's support group on variety of topics[c]	0.72	1.1	2.37	1.3	2.94	1.0
Men's group training[c]	0.50	1.0	1.55	1.3	2.44	1.7
Men's group education[c]	0.54	0.9	1.50	1.1	2.11	1.4
Men's group focused on substance use and mental health[c]	0.61	1.0	1.89	1.1	1.68	1.6
Men's and women's group on training or employment	1.12	1.2	2.06	1.4	1.89	1.7
Men's and women's group on literacy	1.34	1.2	1.89	1.4	2.05	1.5
Health board or policy council	1.65	0.8	1.89	.9	2.05	0.7
Center committees	1.67	1.0	1.94	0.8	2.14	0.9
Men's and women's group on substance use or mental health	1.05	1.1	1.83	1.0	1.42	1.4
Working in the classroom	1.57	1.0	1.89	1.1	2.28	0.9
Dropping off or picking up child from the center	2.20	1.2	2.56	1.3	2.94	1.2
Attending home visits but not participating	2.30	0.8	2.56	0.7	2.32	0.8
Attending home visits and participating	2.11	0.8	2.38	0.8	2.58	0.8
Setting home visit goals	1.94	0.8	2.38	0.9	1.95	0.8
Parent – teacher conferences	1.49	1.2	2.00	1.1	2.11	1.1
Fixing up the center	1.07	1.1	1.33	1.1	1.42	1.5
Sample size	261		18		11	

Note. Early Head Start National Practitioners Survey and the Early Head Start Fatherhood Demonstration Study.

[a]Items were scored as follows: 0 = *no fathers are involved;* 1 = *(a few) up to 20% of fathers;* 2 = *(some) 20% to 50% of fathers;* 3 = *(many) 50% or more;* 4 = *(most) more than 75% of fathers are involved.* The Father Program Activities Scale is the average of all 23 items listed in the table. The Father-Focused Program Activities Scale is the average of 7 items indicated by footnote c.

[b]Four different versions of the survey were administered to Early Head Start directors, fatherhood staff, home visitors and family workers, and teachers. Respondents were asked to report only on father participation in activities that pertained to their work with families. Therefore, not all respondents were asked to report on each listed activity and the number of reporters ranged from 11 to 75.

[c]These seven items make up the Father-Focused Program Activities Scale.

cantly higher at 2.1, showing that up to half of the fathers were involved. On the Father-Focused Program Activities Scale of seven activities explicitly focused on the fathers, the average score of 0.6 showed that these events were likely to be attended by only a very few fathers in the programs (2.0 for mature programs).

Whole family events (e.g., open house or holiday parties) were most popular, followed by group parenting activities, other activities designed to improve parenting, and attending home visits (all averaging 2.3 or higher). However, very few fathers participated in "daddy and me" events, sporting events for fathers, men's groups focused on parenting, or employment services. In mature programs, more than half of the program fathers attended whole-family events as well as socializations (group parent – child events) and other activities designed to improve parenting.

STUDY 2

Sample and Procedures

In February 2001, ACYF partnered with the Office of Child Support Enforcement (OCSE) to fund 21 Early Head Start Fatherhood Demonstration projects for 3 years. The goal of the demonstration was to develop and implement creative practices to increase the involvement of fathers in the Early Head Start program and in the lives of their children. Using their grant funds, programs were expected to hire new fatherhood staff dedicated to reaching out to fathers and to helping design unique services to meet their needs as parents. Each grantee was also expected to partner with its local child support office to offer services that encouraged responsible parenting. Although ACYF provided these basic guidelines, grantees had flexibility in developing their own program goals and service structure.

The findings reported here are based on evaluation data from the 21 demonstration programs over the first 2 years of implementation (2001 – 2003). We use three data sources. First, we conducted two rounds of site visits to the 21 demonstration programs toward the end of their first year (2001 – 2002) and second year (2002 – 2003) of implementation. Second, at the time of the second round of visits, we asked Early Head Start directors, fatherhood staff, home visitors and family workers, and teachers at each participating program to complete a father involvement survey modeled after the instrument used in the National Practitioners Survey. The staff survey achieved an overall response rate of 93% and a 90% response rate among Early Head Start directors. Third, staff members at each program were asked during the second year of the demonstration to report data on the characteristics, involvement, and program participation of the father(s) of each child enrolled in Early Head Start. We collected father data on 1,743 of the 1,871 enrolled children, or 93% of the sample.

Because the demonstration programs were selected through a competitive grant process, they are not necessarily representative of Early Head Start programs nationwide. Compared to programs that responded to the National Practitioners Survey, the demonstration programs more often reported center-based services as their primary program approach and were more likely to serve urban areas (Table 1). A larger proportion of demonstration programs also served predominantly African American or Latin American families.

Results

Comparable to the National Practitioners Study, 47% in the Fatherhood Demonstration Study were resident fathers, and 29% were reported to be involved, nonresident fathers (Table 2). Based on data reported on individual fathers, we also found that 41% of the fathers identified by demonstration staff were married to the child's mother, 26% were unemployed, and 40% had less than a high school education.

Table 2 also shows that nonresident fathers may have been more salient to the demonstration programs than to programs nationally. At the time of the survey, all of the demonstration programs sought to involve resident fathers and father figures in Early Head Start services. The demonstration programs were more likely, however, to attempt to involve fathers who do not live with the enrolled child. Specifically, 95% of demonstration programs targeted nonresident biological fathers compared to 77% nationally, and 84% targeted nonresident father figures compared to only 58% nationally. In addition, a larger fraction of demonstration programs made strong efforts to engage incarcerated fathers.

Next, we explored program involvement. As a result of special programmatic efforts to reach out to men, father involvement often appears higher overall within the demonstration programs compared to programs nationally and to programs ranked at the mature stage of father-friendliness. Among children who had resident fathers, demonstration staff reported that 53% of these fathers participated in at least one program activity and 48% were highly involved with the program. As noted earlier, nationally, 59% of identified resident fathers were reported to have ever participated but only 25% were highly involved. Among nonresident fathers, demonstration staff reported that 45% had participated at least once and 30% were highly involved, compared to 30% and 10% in the national sample, respectively.

Consistent with these results, we found higher father attendance within the demonstration programs when using the same Father Program Activities Scale discussed earlier (Table 3). Specifically, demonstration fathers were much more likely to attend father-focused activities with a Father-Focused Program Activities Scale score of 2.4 compared to 0.6 nationally. Again, these activities include such services as father – child activities, sporting events, men's support groups, and training and education programs for men.

During site visits to the demonstration programs, we found that father-only activities were common. Over time, small groups of committed fathers began participating regularly in peer support groups for men. Nearly all of the demonstration programs offered these groups, adjusting the structure, content, and timing of meetings based on fathers' interests and needs. Staff reported average participation scores of 2.9 for men's groups focused on a range of topics.

Father-only activities, such as sporting events or camping trips, offered additional opportunities for fathers and staff to develop relationships based on mutual trust. Many fathers also sought out employment and training services to help improve their ability to support their children financially. The demonstration programs reported an average participation score of 2.4 for men's groups on training related to employment and 2.1 for men's groups focused on education or literacy, compared to 0.5 for both activities in the national sample. More fathers also appeared to be participating in father-child activities, such as "daddy and me" events and special father – child reading programs, during the second year of the demonstration. The demonstration programs reported participation scores of 2.5 for these activities, compared to 0.8 nationwide. The programs began offering more of these activities as fathers requested and responded to opportunities to bond with their children and families.

Most of the father-focused activities were facilitated by male fatherhood staff hired specifically through the demonstration grant. Fathers reported during focus groups that they appreciated the presence of male staff within the female-dominated environment of Early Head Start. They also felt more comfortable discussing personal issues with a male member of the staff. Teachers and family workers also believed that male staff and highly involved fathers provided good examples for other men and encouraged them to interact in positive and nurturing ways with their small children. Additionally, some demonstration fathers who participated in focus groups reported feeling more welcomed by staff than they had in the past, possibly resulting from extensive staff training on father involvement.

DISCUSSION

This article examined comparable data across two studies, one a survey conducted in 1999 to 2000 of 261 Early Head Start programs, including a subgroup of 18 mature programs with respect to father friendliness, and the other conducted in 2002 to 2003 with a sample of 21 programs participating in a fatherhood demonstration project. In the first study, we found that fathers were becoming involved in programmatic activities, more so in mature programs; from the second study, we learned fathers were even more involved when resources were added through a fatherhood demonstration grant.

Because the same questions were asked, the National Practitioners Survey may be considered a baseline against which progress in demonstration projects as well as future efforts can be tracked. However, the survey achieved only a 63% response rate and probably provides an optimistic assessment of baseline father involvement. Thus, the difference between the results of the two studies here is most likely a conservative estimate of father involvement. On the other hand, we do not know whether reporters in demonstration programs were differentially motivated to report higher levels of father activities, and may have inflated their responses.

The two studies presented in this article demonstrate that a majority of Early Head Start children do have fathers involved in their lives. This finding now has been reported consistently in separate samples of Early Head Start children (ACF, 2002a; Cabrera et al., 2004), Head Start (ACYF, 2002), and other samples of low-income families (Mincy & Oliver, 2003). However, many children live in fragile families, in which fathers are involved but not necessarily living with the child. Interestingly, the two independent programmatic staff samples in this study cited similar overall prevalence of father involvement at 70% to 76% (children with an involved father, whether resident or nonresident), but this is slightly lower than almost 90% by mother report (ACF, 2002a). It is possible that some involved, nonresident fathers may not be salient to intervention program staff and that staff may be underestimating how many fathers are there. Thus, the potential for engaging nonresident involved fathers into program activities may be greater than currently believed to be the case. Others might argue that a father who sees or communicates with a child several times over a 3-month period is not an "involved" father at all. However, for programs serving infants and toddlers, where staff are aware that father presence decreases as children mature (Carlson & McLanahan, 2002), such involvement offers potential for keeping a father in the child's life.

The National Practitioners Survey illustrates the racial and ethnic diversity of fathers in low-income children's families across resident and nonresident status, with attendant implications for programs. A program serving African American families in which a majority of involved fathers is nonresident is likely to use different strategies for engaging fathers than a program serving families with mostly resident fathers.

The ability of national mature programs and fatherhood demonstration programs to engage fathers at intensive levels (participating in the program 3 times a month) is encouraging, given findings from Head Start showing that more intensive father participation in program activities is associated with improved child outcomes (Fagan & Iglesias, 1999) and consistent with studies of father involvement in schools (Nord, Brinhall, & West, 1997).

The program-reported percentage of resident fathers who were "highly involved" was 48%, 40%, and 24% for the demonstration, national mature, and overall national programs, respectively. Comparable figures for nonresident fathers were even more striking at 30%, 14%, and 10%, respectively, and illustrate the potential for engaging involved, nonresident fathers when the resources and focus characteristic of the fatherhood demonstration are applied.

The successes of fatherhood demonstration programs in engaging nonresident fathers and higher scores on the Father-Focused Activities Scale were notable. Activities that were for fathers only were more prevalent in the fatherhood demonstration sites than in mature national sites. However, mature programs versus other national study programs demonstrated more father involvement in parenting education, home visits, and other activities offered to mothers and fathers. The mature father involvement programs in the national study did not have additional Head Start resources for father involvement. Therefore, they appeared to have emphasized involving fathers in the activities they were already offering. The additional resources of the fatherhood demonstration project apparently led to a greater preponderance of activities focused on the men and their personal development (training, education, literacy, support, sports), including potentially resource-intensive efforts to engage nonresident fathers. Thus, two distinct styles of father involvement in Early Head Start appear to be emerging with differing emphases on parenting and men's personal development. A fruitful area for future research will be to explore which combination of approaches leads to greatest gains with respect to the children's development, the ultimate goal of Early Head Start.

The findings presented from these two studies reinforce previous research findings that many fathers are involved in their children's lives, and are getting involved in program activities. As shown by the Fatherhood Demonstration Study, when programs make special efforts to make them feel welcome and create services that meet their needs, fathers appear to respond by participating in larger numbers. Despite these successes, there still are many challenges to full involvement of fathers that need to be overcome. Many programs have still not been successful in engaging large proportions of fathers and father figures in program activities, and it remains to be seen the extent to which father involvement, particularly of nonresident fathers, can be sustained in the absence of special demonstration resources. Findings from this study lay groundwork for probing more deeply into the potential of early intervention, inclusive of fathers.

AFFILIATIONS AND ADDRESSES

Helen H. Raikes, University of Nebraska-Lincoln, 3221 South 76th Street, Lincoln, NE 68506. E-mail: hraikes2@unl.edu. Jeanne Bellotti is at Mathematica Policy Research, Inc.

REFERENCES

Administration for Children and Families. (2002a). *Making a difference in the lives of infants and toddlers and their families.* Washington, DC: Department of Health and Human Services.

Administration for Children and Families. (2002b). *Pathways to quality.* Washington, DC: Department of Health and Human Services.

Administration on Children, Youth and Families. (1999). *Leading the way: Characteristics and early experiences of selected Early Head Start programs. Volume I: Cross site perspectives.* Washington, DC: Department of Health and Human Services.

Administration on Children, Youth and Families. (2000). *Leading the way: Characteristics and early experiences of selected Early Head Start programs. Volume III: Program implementation.* Washington, DC: Department of Health and Human Services.

Administration on Children, Youth and Families. (2002). *A descriptive study of Head Start families: FACES technical report 1.* Washington, DC: Department of Health and Human Services.

Bellotti, J., Vogel, C., Burwick, A., Nagatoshi, C., Ford, M., Schiff, B., et al. (2003). *Dedicated to dads: Lessons from the Early Head Start Fatherhood Demonstration.* Princeton, NJ: Mathematica Policy Research.

Black, M., Dubowitz, H., & Starr, R. H. (1999). African–American fathers in low income, urban families: Development and behavior of their 3-year-old children. *Child Development, 70,* 967–978.

Cabrera, N. J., Ryan, R. M., Shannon, J. D., Brooks-Gunn, J., Vogel, C., Raikes, H., et al. (2004). Low-income fathers' involvement in their toddlers' lives: Biological fathers from the Early Head Start Research and Evaluation study. *Fathering, 2,* 5–20.

Carlson, M., & McLanahan, S. (2002). Fragile families, father involvement and public policy. In C. S. Tamis-LeMonda & N. Cabrera (Eds.), *Handbook of father involvement: Multidisciplinary perspectives.* Mahwah, NJ: Lawrence Erlbaum Associates, Inc.

Cohen, A., & Love, J. (1999). *Fathers are important in Early Head Start.* Unpublished manuscript.

Fagan, J., & Iglesias, A. (1999). Father involvement program effects on fathers, father figures, and their Head Start children: A quasi-experimental study. *Early Childhood Research Quarterly, 14,* 243–269.

Fagan, J., & Palm, G. (2004). *Fathers and early childhood programs.* Clifton Park, NY: Thompson Delmar Learning.

Kitzman, H., Olds, D., Sidora, K., Henderson, C., Hanks, C., Cole, R., et al. (2000). Enduring effects of nurse home visitation on maternal life course: A 3-year follow-up of a randomized trial. *The Journal of the American Medical Association, 283,* 1983–1989.

Mahoney, G., Wiggers, B., & Lash, S. (1996). Using a relationship-focused intervention program to enhance father involvement. *Infant–Toddler Intervention, 6,* 295–308.

McAllister, C. L., Wilson, P. C., & Burton, J. (2004). From sports fans to nurturers: An Early Head Start program's evolution toward father involvement. *Fathering, 2,* 31–60.

Mincy, R. B., & Oliver, H. (2003). *Age, race, and children's living arrangements: Implications for TANF reauthorization* (Policy Brief B–53). Washington, DC: Urban Institute.

Nord, C. W., Brinhall, D., & West, J. (1997). *Fathers' involvement in their children's schools.* Washington, DC: U.S. Department of Education, Office of Educational Research and Improvement.

Raikes, H., Boller, K., van Kammen, W., & Summers, J. (2002). *Father involvement in Early Head Start programs: A practitioners study.* Lincoln: University of Nebraska Press.

Ramey, C. T., & Campbell, F. (1991). Poverty, early childhood education, and academic competence: The Abecedarian experiment. In A. Huston (Ed.), *Children in poverty: Child development and public policy* (pp 190–221). New York: Cambridge University Press.

Tamis-LeMonda, C. S., Shannon, J. D., Cabrera, N., & Lamb, M. (2004). Fathers and mothers at play with their 2 and 3 year olds: Contributions to language and cognitive development. *Child Development, 75,* 1806–1820.

PARENTING: SCIENCE AND PRACTICE
April–September 2006 Volume 6 Numbers 2 & 3 Pages 243–258

Exposure of Low-Income Families and Their Children to Neighborhood Violence and Paternal Antisocial Behavior

Hiram E. Fitzgerald, Lorraine M. McKelvey, Rachel F. Schiffman, and Marcel Montañez

SYNOPSIS

Objective. We examined the relation between neighborhood violence and father antisocial behavior with a national sample of fathers from low-income families with 3-year-old children ***Design.*** Children were classified into 4 groups based on their exposure to father antisocial behavior and neighborhood violence. ***Results.*** Children who experience high levels of each performed more poorly on indicators of emotion regulation. Children in risk groups were exposed to higher levels of family conflict, father depression, and poorer internal and external physical environments than children who were in the low-risk group. Children with fathers who were not antisocial were 3 times more likely to be spanked when the father resided in a high-risk neighborhood. ***Conclusions.*** Fathers should be included in early prevention programs targeting families with very young children, and such programs simultaneously challenged to broaden into community networks.

INTRODUCTION

Low-income children are exposed to higher levels of violence than are children in middle and upper income levels (Evans, 2004; Leventhal & Brooks-Gunn, 2000), including both violence that occurs in the home and in the neighborhood (Chase-Lansdale, Gordon, Brooks-Gunn, & Klebanov, 1997; Cicchetti & Lynch, 1993). Relatively little attention has been paid to differentiating these two sources of violence exposure with respect to child and family functioning. There are well-documented relations between low-income and harsh parenting (Conger & Elder, 1994; Johnson, Cohen, Brown, Smailes, & Bernstein, 1999), familial violence (Sampson, Raudenbush, & Earls, 1997), paternal antisocial behavior (DuRant, Getts, Cadenhead, Emans, & Woods, 1995), substance abuse (Zucker et al., 2000), and poor parent – child relationships (Bradley & Corwyn, 2002, Brooks-Gunn & Duncan, 1997).

Families residing in violent neighborhoods are more likely to be characterized by harsh disciplinary practices than are families that reside in nonviolent neighborhoods (Earls, McGuire, & Shay, 1994). Witnessed or experienced aggression (including childhood maltreatment) during the early childhood years has been linked to heightened behavior problems (Emery & Laumann-Billings, 1988; Kalmuss, 1984; Malinosky-Rummell & Hansen, 1993; Strauss, Gells, & Stienmentz, 1980) and serious mental health problems in victimized children (Bell & Jenkins, 1991; Martinez & Richters, 1993; Osofsky, 2002). Moreover, there is considerable evidence to suggest that poverty exacerbates the level of familial and neighborhood risk to which children are exposed (Evans, 2004), and, in that regard, should be considered to be part of the causal structure that leads to poor developmental outcomes.

One issue to be addressed in this literature is that the characterization of neighborhood or familial violence has been overwhelmingly based on maternal report (Leventhal & Brooks-Gunn, 2000). The Early Head Start Fathers Study provided a unique opportunity to assess neighborhood violence from the father's perspective. Therefore, our first purpose was to assess the impact of neighborhood violence exposure on child and family functioning, with particular emphasis on children's emotional and cognitive functioning. Specifically, we tested the hypothesis that children exposed to high paternal report neighborhood violence would have poorer general functioning than would children residing in less violent neighborhoods.

The historical analysis of the father's role in the family unit provides a framework to guide the systematic study of father's parenting role (Parke, 1995) and his place in the family unit (Loukas, Twitchell, Piejak, Fitzgerald, & Zucker, 1998). Whereas some of this work focused on the positive ways that fathers directly contribute to child development, the dominant view in the literature is that paternal influences on young children are more likely to be indirect via their impact on family functioning and the quality of the mother – child relationship (Lamb, 1987; Parke, 1995). Exceptions to the indirect effects hypothesis are longitudinal studies that focus on the origins of aggression (Huesmann, 1998; Huesmann, Eron, Lefkowitz, & Walder, 1984; Nagin & Tremblay, 2001; Tremblay, 2000) and substance abuse (Fitzgerald, Mun, Zucker, Puttler, & Wong, 2002; Loeber, 1982), which test the hypothesis that paternal antisocial behavior has a direct effect on children and the subsequent intergenerational transmission of aggressive behavior (Fuller et al., 2003; Kwong, Bartholomew, Henderson, & Trinke, 2003). Therefore, the second purpose of this study was to assess the impact of paternal antisocial behavior on child and family functioning, again with particular interest in children's emotional and cognitive functioning (Chase-Lansdale et al., 1997). Specifically, we tested the hypothesis that fathers high in antisocial behavior would be more likely to have children with poorer general functioning than would fathers who were low in antisocial behavior.

Children reared in risky family environments are more likely to have higher levels of hyperactivity and externalizing behavior problems, earlier evidence of negative mood, more problematic social relationships, greater deficits in cognitive functioning, higher levels of aggressive behavior, and more precocious acquisition of cognitive schemas about alcohol and other drugs (Fitzgerald, Davies, & Zucker, 2002; Fitzgerald, Mun, et al., 2002). Moreover, negative parent characteristics such as aggressiveness and antisocial behavior potentiate the appearance of child risk factors. Thus, toddlers high in behavioral undercontrol are likely to show behavioral dysregulation through the elementary years and beyond (Loeber, 1982; Moffitt, 1993). Although biological factors obviously help to account for variation in children's undercontrol, various social and ecological factors contribute to the organization of self-regulation as well, including the social ecology of the neighborhoods that surround many high-risk families (Zucker et al., 2000). These findings suggest that there is a cumulative effect of risk that is particularly devastating to children's cognitive and behavioral development when they reside in chronic poverty (Bradley & Corwyn, 2002; Brooks-Gunn & Duncan, 1997; Evans, 2004; McLoyd, 1998). The third purpose of this study was to assess the combined impact of exposure to risky neighborhood and risky paternal rearing environments on child and family functioning. Specifically, we tested a risk accumulation hypothesis which asserts that children exposed to higher levels of neighborhood violence and higher paternal antisocial behavior will have more emotional and cognitive difficulties than children exposed to less violent rearing environments and less violent fathers.

METHODS

Participants

All men were recruited through the national sample of families participating in the evaluation of Early Head Start Father Involvement with Toddlers Study (FITS; see Boller et al., this issue). For this study, we only included men who were residing in the family home and who were in a romantic relationship with the child's mother when the child was 36 months old ($n = 561$). The final sample used for analyses included 473 resident biological or social fathers who had sufficient data to be classified into risk categories. There were no demographic differences between the 473 men in the analyses and the 88 individuals dropped because missing data precluded classification into risk categories. Ethnically, 45.8% of the fathers were European American, non-Hispanic; 15.9% were African American; 22.8% were Latin American; 4% were distributed among other ethnic groups; and 11.4% did not identify their racial or ethnic tradition. Fathers' average age was 29 years (*range* = 17–58, *SD* = 6.83), and on average had 11.8 years of education (*range* = 1–20, *SD* = 11.05 years). There were nearly equal numbers of boys and girls, and the average age of the children was 40 months (*SD* = 3) at the time that the father interview was completed.

Children were categorized into groups depending on the degree of their exposure to either fathers who scored high in a scale assessing antisocial behavior (Father ASB), a scale assessing paternal reports of the amount of neighborhood violence (Neighborhood Violence), and those exposed to both high-risk conditions, or exposed to neither risk. Neighborhood Violence was defined by fathers' yes – no responses to five questions concerning neighborhood violence: Have you heard or seen a violent crime take place in your neighborhood? Have you known someone who was a victim of a violent crime in your neighborhood? Have you been a victim of a violent crime in your neighborhood? Have you been robbed, mugged, or attacked in the past year? Have you had a relative or close friend in jail? Children whose fathers answered yes to 2 or more of these items were classified as at high risk for exposure to neighborhood violence ($n = 97$) and those whose fathers scored 0 or 1 were scored as at low risk for neighborhood violence ($n = 376$).

Father antisocial behavior was defined by fathers' responses to the following four questions: Have you ever been expelled from school? Have you ever been fired or laid off from a job because of behavior, attitude, or work performance? Have you ever been put in jail, arrested or convicted of a crime, other than drunk driving? Have you ever had a drinking or drug problem or have other people thought you had one? Children whose fathers answered yes to 0 or 1 of these items were classified as at low risk for father antisocial behavior ($n = 324$). Children whose fathers answered affirmatively to 2 or more were classified as at high risk for exposure to father antisocial behavior ($n = 149$).

The use of a criterion of 2 or more to differentiate the samples (rather than the more conventional 3 or more) was dictated by the need to have an adequate number of cases for each of the categories formed based on responses to each of the measures. These categorizations resulted in classifying children into four groups for analyses: low neighborhood violence, low father antisocial behavior (LoNV – LoASB); high neighborhood violence, low father antisocial behavior (HiNV – LoASB); low neighborhood violence, high father antisocial behavior (LoNV – HiASB); and high neighborhood violence, high father antisocial behavior (HiNV – HiASB).

Child Cognitive Measures

Bayley Mental Development Index (MDI). The MDI measures cognitive, language, and social - emotional development. Children were assessed by trained examiners using a standard protocol. The MDI is standardized such that the mean standard score is 100, *SD* = 15.

Puzzle task. During this task, children are asked to solve up to three puzzles of increasing difficulty in 6 to 7 min (Brady-Smith, Ryan, Berlin, Brooks-Gunn, & Fuligni, 2001). Parents are instructed to let their child work on the puzzle independently first, and then to provide assistance. The dyad has up to 4 min to work on each puzzle. Coders reached 85% agreement or higher prior to coding unique interactions. In this study, two scales were used to assess child behavior: Engagement of Parent and Persistence. Engagement of Parent reflects the extent to which the child shows, initiates, or maintains interaction with the parent and communicates positive regard or positive affect to the parent. The focus is on the child's behavior, not the parents. Children are rated from 1 (*very low engagement*) to 7 (*very high engagement*). Persistence measures the degree of goal-orientation, focus, and motivation toward the puzzle throughout the task. Puzzles are challenging and frustrating, thus allowing the assessment of how children persist in their task orientation even when frustrated. Children are rated from 1 (*very low persistence*) to 7 (*very high persistence*). (For additional information about the puzzle task, consult Brooks-Gunn, Liaw, Michael, & Zamsky, 1992.)

Peabody Picture Vocabulary Test. The Peabody Picture Vocabulary Test (PPVT–III) is a measure of receptive vocabulary and a test of verbal ability for ages from 2½ years through adult. The task of the test taker is to select the picture that best represents the meaning of a stimulus word presented orally by the examiner. The PPVT–III was normed on a nationally representative sample of children and adults of various ages so that raw scores can be converted to age-adjusted, standardized scores with a *M* = 100 and a *SD* = 15. All of the examiners were trained to reach at least 85% reliability for administration.

Child Emotion - Behavior Regulation Measures

Bayley Behavior Rating Scale (BRS). The Bayley BRS measures child behavior during MDI administration. It is composed of two subscales: Emotion Regulation (the ability to change tasks with minimal negative affect and the ability to control frustration during task administration) and Orientation – Engagement (the degree of cooperation with the examiner). These ratings are based on a 5-point scale, with 5 indicating the most positive behavior.

Achenbach Child Behavior Check List (CBCL) 2–3 Year Old: Aggression subscale. The CBCL (Achenbach & Rescorla 2000) is completed by each parent independently and provides an assessment of the target child's social and emotional functioning. Adequate construct validity was established by correlations between CBCL scores and scores on a wide range of other measures of child behavior problems. For each of the possible behavior problems, the parent was asked whether the child exhibits this behavior often, sometimes, or never. The Aggression subscale measures 19 aggressive behaviors such as temper tantrums, hitting, and easily frustrated. Scores range from 0 (*not observed* in any item) to 38 (score of 2 *very often true* on every item).

Parent Measures

The Center for Epidemiological Studies-Depression Scale — Short Form [CES-D (SF)]. The CES-D is a 12-item self-report measure of depressive symptoms in community populations (Ross, Murkowski, & Huber, 1983). Respondents were asked the number of days in the past week they had a particular symptom. Symptoms include poor appetite, restless sleep, loneliness, sadness, and lack of energy. Each item is scored on a 4-point Likert-type scale — ranging from 0 (*rarely*) to 3 (*most days*) — indicating the frequency and intensity of the symptom during the previous week.

Parenting Stress Index — Short Form (PSI–SF; Abidin, 1995). Two subscales of the PSI–SF were used: Parental Distress and Parent – Child Dysfunctional Interaction. The 12-item Parental Distress subscale measures the level of distress the parent feels in the role as a parent in relation to personal factors, including a low sense of parental competence, stress related to parenting, depression, and poor social support. The 12-item Parent – Child Dysfunctional Interaction subscale measures the parent's perception that the child does not meet parental expectations and that interactions with the child are not reinforcing to the parent. Responses on the PSI–SF are coded on a 5-point scale, with 5 indicating higher parenting stress.

Family Environment Scale (FES): Family Conflict (Moos & Moos, 1976). The FES measures the social interactions of family members along 10 key dimensions. In this study, the Family Conflict dimension was used. The five Family Conflict items measure the extent of open - expression of anger, aggression, and conflict that characterizes the family. Items rated on a 4-point scale, with 4 indicating high agreement with statements such as the following: "We fight a lot."and "We hardly ever lose our temper."

Parental Modernity Scale (PMS; Schaefer & Edgerton, 1985). Five items collected from the Parental Modernity Scale assessed traditional authoritarian parenting beliefs, with Cronbach's alpha being .76. The scoring of the traditional subscale of the PMS was based on the scales as used in the National Institute of Child Health and Human Development Study of Child Care (ACF, 2002).

Perceived disagreement. The father is asked about much disagreement he and the child's mother have (e.g., none, some, or a great deal) about how the child is reared, how he spends money on the child, how the mother spends money on the child, how much time the father spends with the child, and the father's contribution to child support. Perceived disagreement is the sum score of all six disagreement items. There is a 3-point response range for the items, and as such, the scale range is 0 (*no disagreement*) to 12 (*high disagreement*).

Discipline Severity Index (DSI). The DSI measures the parent's strategies for handling four different potential conflict situations with the child: (1) the child keeps playing with breakable things, (2) the child refuses to eat, (3) the child throws a temper tantrum in a public place, and (4) the child hits the parent in anger. Discipline Severity measures the degree of harshness or discipline strategies reports, on a 1 to 5 scale with 5 indicative of parents who say they would use physical punishment and 1 indicative of parents who would use the mild disciplinary techniques such as time out or removing the child from the situation.

The Early Childhood Home Observation for Measurement of the Environment [(EC) HOME]. The (EC) HOME measures the quality of stimulation and support available to a child in the home environment (Caldwell & Bradley, 1984). For this study, we used a modified version of the instrument (ACF, 2002). The subscales used in the analyses included the Internal Physical Environment subscale to assess the cleanliness, organization, and warmth of the home environment. Items in this subscale are based entirely on interviewer observations during the interview and were each coded on a 3-point scale (scores can range from 3 to 9). We also used the External Physical Environment subscale to measure the external physical environment and living space. Items in this subscale are based entirely on interviewer observations during the interview on aspects of the home's structural safety, adequacy of living space, and quality of outside play environment and street on which the child lives. Each observation was coded on a 3-point scale (scores can range from 5 to 15).

Data Analysis

Hypotheses were tested using multiple analysis of variance (Huberty & Morris, 1989), with Ryan-Holm step-down Šidák adjusted p values (Ludbrook, 1998, 2000), and Šidák adjusted pairwise comparisons. All analyses controlled for key paternal demographic characteristics, including age, education, and ethnicity. Fifty-two children were administered the PPVT in Spanish. However, parsing them into father ASB and neighborhood violence groups resulted in sample sizes as small as 2; therefore, we controlled for ethnicity across all analyses.

RESULTS

Data summarized in Table 1 do not provide support for Hypotheses 1 and 2. There were no differences on any comparison involving children exposed to high neighborhood violence (HiNV – LoASB) and those exposed to low neighborhood violence (LoNV – LoASB), and there weren't any differences on any comparison involving children exposed to high father antisocial behavior (LoNV – HiASB) and those who were not (LoNV – LoASB). However, there was support for the third hypothesis which posited risk cumulation effects on children's general functioning. This was especially evident for behavior regulation (BBRS). Children in the HiNV – HiASB group were significantly poorer in regulatory functioning during administration of the Bayley Scales.

Data summarized in Table 2 support all three hypotheses with respect to the quality of the parenting and home environments differentiating the four children's risk groups. Children in all three risk groups were exposed to greater family conflict than were children in the low-risk group (LoNV – LoASB). Paternal depression, apparently, is related strongly to father antisocial behavior because fathers of children in the HiNV – LoASB group did not significantly differ from the low-risk group, whereas fathers in the

TABLE 1

Early Head Start 36-Month Data: Differences in Children's Behavior as a Function of Neighborhood Risk and Father Risk—Low Neighborhood Violence Exposure, Low Father Antisocial Behavior (LoNV – LoASB); High Neighborhood Violence Exposure, Low Father Antisocial Behavior (HiNV – LoASB); Low Neighborhood Violence Exposure, High Father Antisocial Behavior (LoNV – HiASB); High Neighborhood Violence Exposure, High Father Antisocial Behavior (HiNV – HiASB)

	Children's Risk Groups											
	LoNV – LoASB		HiNV – LoASB		LoNV – HiASB		HiNV – HiASB					
	N	*M*	*N*	*M*	*N*	*M*	*N*	*M*	*F*	*df*	$p^* \leq$	$p^* \leq$
CBCL aggression	248	10.49	46	12.98	90	11.51	48	11.79	2.867	3, 424	.04	*ns*
BBRS: Emotion regulation	222	4.07	46	3.90	81	3.90	46	3.68[a]	4.37	3, 387	.005	.04
Child engagement, mother	220	5.11	45	5.04	76	5.03	39	4.91	.54	3, 372	.654	*ns*
Child persistence, mother	220	4.68	45	4.45	75	4.63	39	4.54	2.57	3, 371	*ns*	*ns*
Child engagement, father	99	5.17	19	5.22	36	5.18	17	5.10	.07	3, 163	*ns*	*ns*
Child persistence, father	99	4.91	19	4.93	36	4.85	17	4.69	.22	3, 163	*ns*	*ns*
Bayley MDI	211	92.53	42	89.80	76	89.27	44	87.95	3.35	3, 365	.07	*ns*
BBRS orientation	223	3.88	46	3.97	81	3.68	46	3.73	2.36	3, 388	.07	*ns*
PPVT standard score	173	86.11	39	83.36	71	84.18	40	79.29	2.03	3, 315	*ns*	*ns*

Note. CBCL = Child Behavior Checklist; MDI = Mental Development Index PPVT = Peabody Picture Vocabulary Test.

$^*p$ = uncorrected p value

p^1 = Ryan-Holm step-down Šidák adjusted p value.

[a]Mean is significantly different from the L - L group at $p < .05$.

[b]Means are significantly different at $p < .05$.

TABLE 2

Early Head Start 36-Month Data: Differences Between Children's Risk Groups as a Function of Parent and Family Characteristics — Risk Groups are Defined by Neighborhood Risk and Father Risk: Low Neighborhood Violence Exposure, Low Father Antisocial Behavior (LoNV – LoASB); High Neighborhood Violence Exposure, Low Father Antisocial Behavior (HiNV – LoASB); Low Neighborhood Violence Exposure, High Father Antisocial Behavior (LoNV – HiASB); High Neighborhood Violence Exposure, High Father Antisocial Behavior (HiNV – HiASB)

	Children's Risk Groups											
	LoNV – LoASB		HiNV – LoASB		LoNV – HiASB		HiNV - HiASB					
	N	*M*	*N*	*M*	*N*	*M*	*N*	*M*	*F*	*df*	$p^* \leq$	$p^1 \leq$
FES family conflict	247	1.35	47	1.58[a]	90	1.56[a]	47	1.56[a]	7.45	3, 423	.001	.001
PSI parent distress	250	18.66	46	20.33	90	20.01	48	20.72	3.17	3, 426	.02	ns
PSI parent – child dysfunction	248	14.08	47	14.54	90	14.42	48	14.84	.62	3, 425	ns	ns
CES depression father	248	3.46	47	5.39	90	5.91[a]	48	7.25[a]	12.28	3, 425	.001	.001
Disagree/conflict with mother	249	1.45	47	1.99	90	1.97	48	1.75	1.58	3, 426	ns	ns
Parent modernity: Traditional	244	15.03	46	15.03	89	15.35	48	15.94	1.57	3, 419	ns	ns
Discipline severity index	250	3.23	47	3.63	90	3.85	48	3.43	2.88	3, 427	ns	ns
Internal physical environment	220	8.12	43	7.51	79	7.50[a]	44	7.43[a]	6.47	3, 378	.001	.001
External physical environment	220	12.72	43	11.62[a]	78	12.39[b]	45	11.14[a,b]	8.62	3, 380	.001	.001

Note. FES = Family Environment Scale; PSI = Parenting Stress Index; CES = Center for Epidemiological Studies.
$^*p$ = uncorrected p value
p^1 = Ryan-Holm step-down Šidák adjusted p.
[a]Mean is significantly different from the L-L group at $p < .05$.
[b]Means are significantly different at $p < .05$.

HiNV – HiASB group and the LoNV – HiASB group did differ from the LoNV – LoASB group. The quality of the internal and external characteristics of the home environments differed for children as a result of group membership. Characteristics of the internal physical environment appear to relate to father antisocial behavior, as the same pattern of significant differences that was demonstrated with paternal depression were evidenced. However, qualities of the external rearing environment appear to depend on neighborhood quality, as children in the LoNV – HiASB group did not differ from children in the LoNV – LoASB group with respect to the quality of the external home environment.

Although Parental Distress and DSI were only nonsignificant trends after correcting for multiple analyses, we were prompted to examine spanking as a disciplinary technique for two main reasons. First, the national evaluation of Early Head Start suggested that fathers of Early Head Start children were less likely to spank their children than were fathers in the comparison groups (ACF, 2002), and second, spanking is a direct and felt form of aggression and violence from the child's point of view. We used odds ratios to predict whether children in the four groups were differentially at risk for being spanked. Children exposed to high neighborhood violence were 1.9 ($p < .05$) times more likely to be spanked than were children exposed to low neighborhood violence; children exposed to fathers high in antisocial behavior were 1.3 (*ns*) times more likely to be spanked than were children exposed to low father antisocial behavior. The odds ratios examining the moderating effects of father antisocial behavior demonstrated that children living with fathers high in antisocial behavior are equally likely to be spanked (odds = 1.4, *ns*) regardless of the risk present in the neighborhood. However, for children living with fathers who scored low on antisocial behavior, the risk of being spanked increased 3.25 ($p < .05$) times when the father was living in a high-risk neighborhood (see Table 3).

DISCUSSION

The dominant characterization is that the vast majority of fathers participating in FITS do not report residing in violent neighborhoods, being engaged in high levels of antisocial behavior, or viewing their marital and family environments as problematic. For children reared in such environments, there are no a priori reasons to suspect that such factors differentially contribute to risky outcomes such as aggression and antisocial behavior. Nevertheless, the negative consequences of poverty for many low-income children have been thoroughly documented (Evans, 2004), as has evidence for risk aggregation (Fitzgerald, Mun, et al., 2002), so even

TABLE 3
Odds of Being Spanked as a Function of High or Low Exposure to Neighborhood Violence and Paternal Antisocial Behavior

		Spanking					
		Yes		No			
Father ASB	Neighborhood	*n*	%	*n*	%	Odds	Odds Ratio
HiASB	HiNV	18	3.8	30	6.3	0.60	1.14
	LoNV	41	8.7	60	12.7	0.68	
LoASB	HiNV	28	5.9	21	4.4	1.33	
	LoNV	80	16.9	195	41.2	0.41	3.25*

Note. ASB = antisocial behavior; HiASB = high ASB; HiNV = high neighborhood violence; LoNV = low neighborhood violence; LoASB = low ASB.
*$p < .05$.

children in the LoNV – LoASB group may be at risk for various aspects of cognitive development, school achievement, and social - emotional functioning (Evans, 2004) when compared to children residing in high socioeconomic households.

Children in this study who were exposed to high levels of neighborhood violence and father antisocial behavior evidenced poorer emotion regulation. This domain of child behavior has been repeatedly demonstrated to characterize young children at risk for subsequent antisocial behavior, substance abuse, delinquency, and poor academic achievement, with accumulating evidence for intergenerational transmission of such negative consequences (Doumas, Margolin, & John, 1994; Fuller et al., 2003). What is striking about this data is the impact of neighborhood violence exposure to the early differentiation of risk for low-income children.

These findings are consistent with numerous reports detailing the broad "causal" contributions of poverty to poor human functioning (Brooks-Gunn & Duncan, 1997; Evans, 2004), particularly in high-technology societies. Moreover, they suggest that early prevention programs such as Early Head Start must attend to an extremely broad set of developmental issues in efforts to provide more optimal experiential environments for children. Providing home visiting to enhance maternal caregiving skills may be ineffective if the child also is routinely exposed to high family conflict, harsh paternal parenting, and psychopathology (depression and antisocial behavior) embedded within the context of a violent neighborhood. These findings provide additional support for proponents of comprehensive and systemic models of early intervention that focus on individual development only in the context of change models that include family dynamics, community networking, and community change (Cicchetti & Lynch, 1993). More importantly, they provide evidence that fathers must be part of the equation used to assess parental influences on child development if such programs are to succeed.

AFFILIATIONS AND ADDRESSES

Hiram E. Fitzgerald, University Outreach and Engagement, Kellogg Center, Garden Level, Michigan State University, East Lansing, MI 48824. E-mail: fitzger9@msu.edu. Lorraine M. McKelvey is at the University of Arkansas for Medical Sciences. Rachel F. Schiffman is at the University of Wisconsin, Milwaukee. Marcel Montañez is at New Mexico State University.

ACKNOWLEDGMENTS

Portions of this article were presented at the biennial meetings of the World Association for Infant Mental Health, Australia, 2004; the International Society on Infant Studies, Chicago, 2004; and the Society for Research on Child Development, June, 2003. Research reported herein was supported in part by Grant 90YF0010 from the Administration for Children, Youth, and Families Department of Health and Human Services to H. E. Fitzgerald and R. F. Schiffman, and by Michigan State University, Office of the Assistant Provost for Outreach and Engagement. Preparation of the article was also supported by Grant R37 AA0705–16 (R. A. Zucker and H. E. Fitzgerald) from the National Institute of Alcohol Abuse and Alcoholism.

REFERENCES

Abidin, R. R. (1995). *Parenting Stress Index* (3rd ed.). Odessa, FL: Psychological Assessment Resources.

Achenbach, T. M., & Rescorla, L.A. (2000). *Manual for the ASEBA Preschool Forms and Profiles.* Burlington: University of Vermont Department of Psychiatry.

Administration for Children and Families. (2002). *Making a difference in the lives of infants and toddlers and their families. The impact of Early Head Start.* Washington, DC: Department of Health and Human Services.

Bell, C. C., & Jenkins, E. J. (1991). Traumatic stress and children. *Journal of Health Care for the Poor and Underserved, 2,* 175–185.

Bradley, R. H., & Corwyn, R. F. (2002). Socioeconomic status and child development. *Annual Review of Psychology, 53,* 371–399.

Brady-Smith, C., Ryan, R. M., Berlin, L. J., Brooks-Gunn, J., & Fuligni, A. S. (2001). *36-month child–parent interaction rating scales for the puzzle task assessment.* New York: Early Head

Start Research and Evaluation Project, Center for Children and Families, Teachers College, Columbia University.

Brooks-Gunn, J., & Duncan, G. (1997). The effects of poverty on children. *The Future of Children, Children and Poverty, 7,* 55–71.

Brooks-Gunn, J., Liaw, F., Michael, A., & Zamsky, E. (1992). *Manual for coding the puzzle task.* Newark Observational Study of the Teenage Parent Demonstration Project.

Caldwell, B. M., & Bradley, R. H. (1984). *Home observation for measurement of the environment.* Little Rock: University of Arkansas.

Chase-Lansdale, P. L., Gordon R. A., Brooks-Gunn, J., & Klebanov, P. K. (1997). Neighborhood and family influences on the intellectual and behavioral competence of preschool and early school-age children. In J. Brooks-Gunn, G. J. Duncan, & J. L. Aber (Eds.). *Neighborhood poverty. Vol. 1. Context and consequences for children* (pp. 79–118). New York: Russell Sage Foundation.

Cicchetti, D., & Lynch, M. (1993). Toward an ecological/transactional model of community violence and child maltreatment: Consequences for children's development. *Psychiatry, 56,* 96–118.

Conger, R. D., & Elder, H., Jr. (1994). *Families in troubled times.* New York: Aldine de Gruyter.

Doumas, D., Margolis, G., & John, R. S. (1994). Intergenerational transmission of aggression across three generations. *Journal of Family Aggression, 9,* 157–175.

DuRant, R. H., Getts, A., Cadenhead, C., Emans, S. J., & Woods, E. R. (1995). Exposure to violence and victimization and depression, hopelessness, and purpose in life among adolescents living in and around public housing. *Developmental and Behavioral Pediatrics, 16,* 233–237.

Earls, F., McGuire, J., & Shay, S. (1994). Evaluating a community intervention to reduce the risk of child abuse: Methodological strategies in conducting neighborhood surveys. *Child Abuse and Neglect, 18,* 473–485.

Emery, R. E., & Laumann-Billings, L. (1988). An overview of the nature, causes and consequences of abusive family relationships. *American Psychologist, 53,* 121–135.

Evans, G. W. (2004). The environment of childhood poverty. *American Psychologist, 59,* 77–92.

Fitzgerald, H. E., Davies, W. H., & Zucker, R. A. (2002). Growing up in an alcoholic family: Structuring pathways for risk aggregation and theory-driven intervention. In R. J. McMahon & R. DeV. Peters (Eds.), *The effects of parental dysfunction on children* (pp. 127–1146). New York: Kluwer.

Fitzgerald, H. E., Mun, E. Y., Zucker, R A, Puttler, L. I., & Wong, M. M. (2002). Pathways to alcoholism during infancy and early childhood. In H. E. Fitzgerald, K. Karraker, & T. Luster (Eds.), *Infant development: Ecological perspectives* (pp. 221–252). New York: Routledge/Falmer Press.

Fuller, B. E., Chermack, S. T., Cruise, K. A., Kirsch, E., Fitzgerald, H. E., & Zucker, R. A. (2003). Predictors of childhood aggression across three generations in children of alcoholics: Relationships involving parental alcoholism, individual and spousal aggression, and parenting practices. *Journal of Studies on Alcohol, 64,* 472–483.

Huberty, C. J., & Morris, J. D. (1989). Multivariate analysis versus multiple univariate analyses. *Psychological Bulletin, 105,* 302–308.

Huesmann, L. R. (1998). The role of social information processing and cognitive schema in the acquisition and maintenance of habitual aggressive behavior. In R. E. Geen & E. Donerstein (Eds.), *Human aggression: theories, research, and implications for policy* (pp. 73–109). New York: Academic.

Huesmann, L. R., Eron, L. D., Lefkowitz, M. M., & Walder, L. O. (1984). Stability of aggression over time and generations. *Developmental Psychology, 20,* 1120–1134.

Johnson, J. G., Cohen, P., Brown, J., Smailes, E. M., & Bernstein, D. P. (1999). Childhood maltreatment increases risk for personality disorders during early childhood. *Archives of General Psychiatry, 56,* 600–606.

Kalmuss, D. S. (1984). The intergenerational transmission of marital aggression. *Journal of Marriage and the Family, 46,* 11–19.

Kwong, M. J., Bartholomew, K., Henderson, A. J. Z., & Trinke, S. J. (2003). The intergenerational transmission of relationship violence. *Journal of Family Psychology, 17,* 288–301.

Lamb, M. E. (1987). *The father's role: Cross-cultural perspectives.* Hillsdale, NJ: Lawrence Erlbaum Associates, Inc.

Leventhal, T., & Brooks-Gunn, J. (2000). The neighborhoods they live in: The effects of neighborhood residence on child and adolescent outcomes. *Psychological Bulletin, 126,* 309–337.

Loeber, R. (1982). The stability of antisocial and delinquent child behavior: A review. *Child Development, 53,* 1431–1446.

Loukas, A., Twitchell, G. R., Piejak, L. A., Fitzgerald, H. E., & Zucker, R. A. (1998). The family as a unity of interacting personalities. In L. L'Abate (Ed.), *Handbook of family psychopathology* (pp. 35–59). New York: Guilford.

Ludbrook, J. (1998). Multiple comparison procedures updated. *Clinical and Experimental Pharmacology and Physiology, 25,* 1032–1037.

Ludbrook, J. (2000). Multiple inferences using confidence intervals. *Clinical and Experimental Pharmacology and Physiology, 27,* 212–215.

Malinosky-Rummell, R., & Hansen, D. J. (1993). Long-term consequences of childhood physical abuse. *Psychological Bulletin, 114,* 68–79.

Martinez, P., & Richters, J. E. (1993). The NIMH Community Violence Project: II. Children's distress symptoms associated with violence exposure. *Psychiatry: Interpersonal and Biological Processes, 56,* 22–35.

McLoyd, V. C. (1998). Socioeconomic disadvantage and child development. *American Psychologist, 53,* 185–204.

Moffitt, T. E. (1993). "Life-course-persistent" and "adolescent-limited" antisocial behaviour: A developmental taxonomy. *Psychological Review, 100,* 674–701.

Moos, R., & Moos, B. S. (1976). A typology of family social environments. *Family Process, 15,* 357–371.

Nagin, D. S., & Tremblay, R. E. (2001). Parental and early childhood predictors of persistent physical aggression in boys from kindergarten to high school. *Archives of General Psychiatry, 58,* 389–394.

Osofsky, J. D. (2002). The effects of exposure to violence on infants: Current perspectives and directions for the future. In H. E. Fitzgerald, K. H. Karraker, & T. Luster (Eds.), *Infant development: Ecological perspectives* (pp. 252–271). New York: Routledge/Falmer.

Parke, R. D. (1995). Fathers and families. In M. H. Bornstein (Ed.), *Handbook of parenting. Vol. 3: Status and social conditions of parenting* (pp. 27–63). Mahwah, NJ: Lawrence Erlbaum Associates, Inc.

Ross, C. E., Mirowsky, J., & Huber, J. (1983). "Dividing work, sharing work, and in-between: Marriage patterns and depression." *American Sociological Review, 48,* 809–823.

Sampson, R. J., Raudenbush, S. W., & Earls, F. (1997). Neighborhoods and violent crime: A multilevel study of collective efficacy. *Science, 277,* 918–924.

Schaefer, E. S., & Edgerton, M. (1985). Parent and child correlates of parental modernity. In I. Sigel (Ed.), *Parental belief systems* (pp. 287–318). New York: Lawrence Erlbaum Associates, Inc.

Strauss, M, A, Gells, R. J., & Stienmentz, S. K. (1980). *Behind closed doors: Violence in the American family.* Garden City, NY: Anchor.

Tremblay, R. E. (2000). The development of aggressive behavior during childhood: What have we learned in the past century? *International Journal of Behavioral Development, 24,* 129–141.
Zucker, R. A., Fitzgerald, H. E., Refior, S. K., Puttler, L. I., Pallas, D. M., & Ellis, D. A. (2000). The clinical and social ecology of childhood for children of alcoholics: Description of a study and implications for a differentiated social policy. In H. E. Fitzgerald, B. M. Lester, & B. Zuckerman (Eds.), *Children of addiction: Research, health, and policy issues* (pp. 109–142). New York: Garland.

PARENTING: SCIENCE AND PRACTICE
April–September 2006 Volume 6 Numbers 2 & 3 Pages 259–271

Lessons Learned from Early Head Start for Fatherhood Research and Program Development

Robert H. Bradley, Jeffrey K. Shears, Lori A. Roggman, and Catherine S. Tamis-LeMonda

SYNOPSIS

This Special Issue presents a series of studies on men who functioned as fathers in the Early Head Start National Evaluation Study. The pieces focused on how these men viewed themselves as fathers, what they did with and for their children, how that mattered in the lives of children, and what Early Head Start programs were doing to try to foster positive involvement of fathers in the lives of their children. This final article reflects on those efforts and tries to place them in the broader literature on family life among the poor and governmental efforts to assist those families. Special attention is given to the complexity of family life in the 21st century and to the challenges that face men who are often trying to parent in highly uncertain and unstable conditions.

INTRODUCTION

In this Special Issue of *Parenting: Science and Practice*, we have presented a set of interrelated studies conducted by the Father Studies Workgroup of the Early Head Start Research Consortium. The focus was on fathers of infants who are living in circumstances of poverty. These studies arose out of our commitment to understanding fathers' early influences in children's lives as well as the value of Early Head Start as an intervention to support families in promoting the optimal development of their infants and toddlers. Furthermore, we wanted to take advantage of this opportunity to study fathers from diverse cultures and circumstances in multiple regions of the United States.

Our hope in the father studies component of the National Early Head Start Research and Evaluation Project was to try to better understand the men who were functioning as fathers to Early Head Start children, how they thought of themselves as fathers, what they did with and for their children, what kinds of relationships they formed with their children, how the characteristics of the men themselves and the context of parenting affected what they did and the quality of those relationships, and how the behavior of fathers mattered in the lives of the children. It is to those ends that the particular studies represented in this Special Issue were directed. Using various research methods (quantitative and qualitative as well as observed and self-reported) with diverse samples (urban, rural, multiple ethnicities), the studies presented in this Special Issue fall into three broad categories: fathers' involvement with their children, paternal influence on children's development, and fathers' participation in Early Head Start programs.

It was partly because of the rapidly changing world of family life that the father studies component of the Early Head Start National Evaluation Study was initiated. In these circumstances, men with limited resources who are uncertain of the future are particularly challenged to identify precisely the role they should play in the lives of their children. Likewise, society as a whole is being challenged to construct a clear, consistent, and productive perspective on low-income fathers. On the one side, there is a recurrent belief that fathers are important to family life and child well-being and that society should do its utmost to support men in their roles as fathers. On the other side, there is a belief that men have become marginal members of families and are often detrimental to family functioning (e.g., deadbeat dads, abusive fathers, inconsistent parenting), and that society should simply force these fathers to pay their fair share of financial support for children.

A systems view of family life and child development led us to believe that clearly defined roles for fathers and tight connections between what fathers do and how children function would not likely emerge for families that are attempting to confront adversity and instability with limited resources. Neither did it seem likely that social institutions could readily provide the kinds of supports needed to quickly change the balance in favor of productive engagements and strong positive impacts. It is not surprising, then, that there is a sense of inchoate purpose expressed by many men in the article by Summers, Boller, Schiffman, and Raikes (this issue). Men clearly want to "be there" for their children and for their families, but they are sometimes hard pressed to specify exactly what being there means in terms of activities, behaviors, and contributions to family life. The voices describing their experiences and perceptions of "good fathering" highlight four major roles: stability, teaching, physical interaction, and emotional support. Evidence from other survey studies indicates that fathers, on average, spend relatively modest amounts of time with their children and that mothers retain the lion's share of responsibility for most things pertaining to children (excepting financial responsibility; Hofferth, Stueve, Pleck, Bianchi, & Sayer, 2002). Accordingly, it is perhaps not surprising that no matter how the researchers in this Special Issue attempted to classify fathers, by behavior or by relationship, no single pattern emerged as predominant. This diffusion of paternal roles and responsibilities is one reason that family scholars have become skeptical about the value of equating the sheer amount of time fathers spend with children or the exact nature of their activities as evidence of the quality of their involvement (Lamb, 2000; Parke, 2002). Good fathering could entail quite different sets of activities and even quite varied amounts of time in different families and communities.

FATHERS' INVOLVEMENT AND INFLUENCE

A major goal of the father's component of the Early Head Start national evaluation study was to explicate how low-income fathers matter in the lives of their children. This has proven no mean feat as it has been devilishly difficult to construct a system for precisely classifying the nature of participating fathers' relationships to child and family — good explanatory science benefits from precise classification of those factors and processes one wants to explain. The report by Vogel, Bradley, Raikes, Boller, and Shears (this issue) brings to mind the difficulty of classifying the exact nature of men's connections to their children and families. Fathers' relationships and proximity to their children and their children's mothers were diverse and often unstable. The diversity of relationships between fathers and other family members who participated in the Early Head Start National Evaluation Study, and the instability present in many homes, may have led to a less consistent organization of parenting behavior among Early Head Start fathers than is often seen in studies of middle-class parents.

Fathers' own descriptions of involvement with their children indicate a great deal of variability in how low-income men focus their parenting role (Summers et al., this issue). The report by Ryan, Martin, and Brooks-Gunn (this issue) shows that, although mothers' parenting and fathers' parenting tend to be organized similarly, the connections among various aspects of parenting behavior are tighter for mothers than fathers. The study by Shannon, Tamis-LeMonda, and Cabrera (this issue) likewise found that the factor structure of paternal behavior accounted for less than 50% of the variance when children were 6 months old and barely more than one third of the variance when children were 14 months old. These findings are predictable from dynamic systems theory. Specifically, if one assumes that men's roles as parents are not strongly and consistently prescribed and supported within a society, then their behavior as parents is unlikely to be tightly organized around a small number of central "attractors" (to use dynamic systems terminology). The links to attractors such as nurturer or teacher, for example, might be less strong than is the case for mothers. As well, for fathers there may be additional attractors (e.g., buddy, liaison) depending on context and circumstances. When disturbances to the father's life or the family system occur (or even just at the point of developmental transitions for the child), it is likely that fathers' behavior will become disorganized temporarily, only to gradually reorganize around a new set of attractors. Previous studies have shown that paternal behavior is multidimensional rather than being tightly organized around a small number of central roles (Bader, 1995; England & Folbre, 2002; Graham & Beller, 2002; Lamb, 2002; Palkovitz, 2002; Rodhalm & Larson 1982).

The contributions of fathers to infant development also appear to be somewhat less consistent than is the case for mothers. Similar to much father research over the last few decades, the results of studies reported in this Special Issue suggest that, although fathers may play an important role in early infant development, their contributions often appear less direct than the contributions of mothers (Lamb, 1997; Yogman, 1981). In both the Ryan et al. (this issue) and Shannon et al. (this issue) studies, positive fathering behaviors were associated with positive child functioning; but the amount of variance accounted for was relatively small. In the Ryan et al. study (this issue), the data suggest that the same parenting behaviors in fathers and mothers contribute to child outcomes, yet fathers may have less of an impact. However, it would be a mistake, based on such findings, to conclude that fathers do not matter that much in the lives of low-income children. Rather, the principles of dynamic systems theory would suggest that researchers carefully examine the conditions impinging on father and family and not generalize findings across developmental domains or even across developmental periods within domains. In some cases, "effects" are likely to be more pronounced when the overall system is in a highly stable state and when there is tight alignment of system components directed toward a particular end state. In other cases, powerful effects emerge as a by-product of major shifts or realignments within systems—what did not matter before the transition suddenly matters a lot. Finally, it is important to remember the "butterfly" effect; that is, a small action at one point in time and space starts a process that results in considerable change somewhere downstream (e.g., dad reading to a 3-year-old may have only a marginal impact on early literacy but a much more pronounced impact on college success).

The failure to observe consistent, strong connections between what fathers do and children's adaptive functioning in the studies included in this

Special Issue may also be due to the diversity of participants in the Early Head Start national evaluation sample. Evidence of fathers' contributions to infant development has more consistently emerged in studies of European American middle-class intact families in which the fathers are traditional residential biological fathers (Vogel et al., this issue); that is, in generally more stable, well buttressed systems as predicted by systems theory. The fathers enrolled in the Early Head Start study were, by contrast, mostly low-income ethnic and racial minorities, and many were nonresidential or social father figures. Such men are often less well connected to and less well supported by the larger communities in which they reside and the social and economic institutions of those communities. Results from the study by Vogel and colleagues (this issue) suggest that children residing with a biological father score higher on developmental indicators, but this pattern was consistent only for European Americans. Inconsistent findings among African American and Latin American fathers suggest possible different dynamics in those groups that should be examined further.

In complex systems such as families, important functional relations can be difficult to detect. Accordingly, it was especially significant that evidence of a complex relation emerged in the report by Ryan et al. (this issue). Their investigation was aimed at answering questions such as "Can one parent's positive attitude and behavior counter the negative attitude and behavior of the other parent? Or, do children with two positive parents display higher levels of positive responses than children from mixed dyad or two negative parents?" The answers to these questions, according to Ryan et al., suggest that the presence of two positive parents contributes more to child well-being than when one parent displays a negative parenting style, regardless of which parent it is. Father presence thus had a similar effect on the child to mother presence, providing a partial counter to findings that the amount of variance in child outcomes explained by mothers' behavior is greater than the amount attributable to fathers' behavior. Even so, the overall impact of fathers' behavior was modest. From the vantage point of systems theory, such small effects are not surprising. In simple systems, powerful effects of one system element on another are commonplace. By contrast, in complex systems (such as is the case for most low-income families living in America), large effects are rarely observed.

Several factors likely contribute to the relatively modest observed association between paternal behavior and children's early development. First, fathers on average spend less time with children than do mothers, so if a kind of dose-response effect operates for any particular type of parenting behavior, one would anticipate a smaller father effect (Hofferth et al., 2002). Second, the effect of any particular parenting behavior is partly determined by the overall context of parenting and home life in which it is embedded (Darling & Steinberg, 1993). If one positive aspect of parenting behavior frequently co-occurs with other good or mutually supportive types of parenting behavior, the greater the likely impact connected to the former (and the same is true for mutually occurring bad behaviors). Because there is a higher degree of co-occurrence among good behaviors for mothers, a tighter alignment of positive parenting behaviors, the likelihood of significant impact for mothers is greater. Third, there is greater likelihood of significant impact if behavior is stable through time (Bloom, 1964). As the study by Shannon et al. (this issue) shows, there is only modest stability of father behavior across time and no predictability from 6-month father behavior to 14-month child behavior. Together, these factors suggest that less time spent with the child + less consistency or alignment of father behaviors within time + less stability over time = less impact on the child. These general principles accepted, it would be a mistake to apply them too readily to everything pertaining to low-income fathers. In complex, dynamic systems, it is not unusual for "effects" to be disproportionate to inputs from specific system components.

FATHERS' PARTICIPATION IN EARLY HEAD START

The article by Raikes and Bellotti (this issue) indicates that Head Start and Early Head Start agencies, although they have a long history of working with poor families, are struggling to figure out how to engage poor fathers. A majority of the children enrolled in Early Head Start had a father or father-figure, and the majority of these fathers or father-figures were residing with the child, but fathers remained noticeably less involved than mothers in most programs. Historically, institutions focused on involving parents were mostly trying to involve mothers. This focus on mothers could be explained partly by the socially accepted parenting role. Recent shifts in fathering roles, as highlighted by Summers et al. (this issue), suggests a move from a more traditional role toward a more contemporary fathering role that is complex and dynamic. In response, Early Head Start programs are attempting to provide services and activities to increase father participation in the program. Unfortunately, there is yet no clear road map to help set directions; and even the most mature programs (in terms of working with fathers) have yielded only modest success. Such findings are not surprising. Most efforts by social and governmental institutions to engage and support fathers have been only marginally successful.

There is, at best, only a loose connection between most low-income men and the social institutions involved with the care of children (churches are perhaps something of an exception; Mincy & Pouncy, 2002). There is a long history of mutual disregard. Accordingly, the beliefs, goals, and practices of many institutions are not aligned with the habits, dispositions, and needs of fathers. Neither is in good position to be maximally supportive of the other, meaning that the desires of individual men to "be there" in some positive way for their children may not be promoted to any great degree by most social institutions as they currently operate. But the information contained in the Raikes and Bellotti (this issue) article also contains seeds of optimism, suggesting that Early Head Start programs are moving along a track that is connecting them more to the needs of low-income men — albeit slowly. The Early Head Start father-involvement demonstration programs, funded specifically to increase father involvement, were more successful in involving all fathers, especially nonresidential fathers, than the Early Head Start programs in the national study. Having male staff members, particularly a father involvement coordinator, was characteristic of programs with greater father participation. The role models male staff members provide may be especially important to young fathers with little prior experience with children or to those who lacked a father or father-figure growing up.

Other findings from the studies reported in this Special Issue may inform productive program practice for institutions, such as Head Start, interested in successfully engaging fathers. The first recommendation is that almost assuredly a "one size fits all" model is not likely to be the most productive way to gain meaningful participation from fathers. Rather than a rigid procedure for intervention approaches to father involvement, programs are likely to benefit from a more open-ended approach that allows flexibility in services depending on family structure, relationships, and culture. Not only does the Vogel et al. (this issue) study show that there is a diversity of relationships between father-figures and their children and families, but it also shows that those patterns of relationships are associated with child outcomes differentially depending on ethnic group. No single template for what to focus on or how to focus on it emerges about relationships between father and child. Likewise, the studies by Shannon et al. (this issue), Ryan et al. (this issue), and Fitzgerald, McKelvey, Schiffman, & Montañez (this issue) show that some low-income fathers play against type; that is, they are very stimulating and also very responsive to their children. Generally, competent fathers may be interested in some targeted skill-building classes pertaining to certain aspects of parenting, but may not be good candidates for the omnibus, packaged "good parenting practices" class. Programs involving fathers of young infants should benefit from understanding why fathers are involved in their child's life and the various types of involvement that are valued by individual fathers as important to being a "good father."

The findings by Ryan et al. (this issue) further suggest that it may be important to understand more about coparenting and what the mother is doing as well to provide effective early interventions that involve fathers. The study by Fitzgerald et al. (this issue), addressing neighborhood violence and fathers' antisocial behaviors as they interact to affect children's development, particularly reveals the need to individualize programming for fathers. Their study shows that fathers struggle more and parent less well when they live in violent neighborhoods; but that fathers' responses to violence depends on their own level of antisocial behavior. When children are exposed both to violence and to their fathers' antisocial behaviors, such as drug use or being arrested, the children have lower scores on emotional regulation and cognitive functioning. These findings suggest that prevention programs in poor economic areas should involve fathers as part of the intervention if there are to be optimal effects on child outcomes. The pattern of supports needed, and the focus of intervention needed, are likely to be different depending on both community factors and the father's own personality. These findings, although again not surprising in light of the broader literature showing that both parental personality and family context affect parenting, may help to identify key aspects of community conditions and parental personality in need of more flexible and creative approaches by social institutions such as Early Head Start.

Results from the studies reported by Raikes and Bellotti (this issue), together with findings from other studies, suggest that service agencies may need to have a rather broad package of possible service options available and that any "core" program should be rather slim and basic. The results reported by Raikes and Bellotti intimate that the core should perhaps focus on social network building. The diversity of fathers and families also suggests that the core should perhaps include a family assessment, which is followed either by individually father-prescribed activities or by program components selected from a rather broad menu of options (based on the capacity of the agency to offer such an array of options). Given the general lack of connection between fathers and social institutions and the various stresses on family life, it may be better that most core interventions be brief, followed by additional components selected at the father's and family's discretion. Interventions for fathers may work best when they remain flexible and ready to take advantage of opportunities as they present themselves.

Findings from the practitioners' study lead to another recommendation for social agencies: namely, they may wish to use a different pitch with fathers than would typically be used with mothers. It is not that mothers and fathers have entirely different agenda for their children, but mothers tend to be more tightly focused on addressing immediate needs, a focus which is largely aligned with program agenda for most early childhood agencies. Fathers, by contrast, have agenda that are somewhat more distal and long term. In the Summers et al. (this issue) piece, fathers talked about their role as exposing children to the world, inculcating social values, being a good "role model," and building self-reliance and even a work ethic. Finding ways to connect to these agenda and presenting ideas and activities that seem to support such proclivities may find fathers more willing partners in common enterprises. To be a bit more concrete, some fathers may be less interested in learning to be sensitive than in learning techniques for fostering self-respect and self-reliance — although those techniques may involve being sensitive enough to help children learn to self-regulate.

METHODS FOR STUDYING FATHERS

Our attempts to meet these challenges in a large-scale, multisite study were unprecedented when we began, but have since influenced other large-scale studies to attempt large-scale studies of low-income fathers (Three City Study, 2006). The research reported in this Special Issue began with well-developed "tight" methods developed over many decades for studying mothers, but then also included newer, less well-developed techniques to explore other aspects of father behavior and to ask fathers more directly about their experiences as fathers and their reflections about their roles and their involvement with their children, and to observe them in less structured situations.

One of our first methodological challenges was recruitment and retention. Our researchers followed fathers through the eyes of their children, therefore identifying a man "most like a father" to the child when the child's biological father was not involved. This approach is unlike that of policy researchers who have tracked biological fathers over time to see when fathers stay and when they leave in relation to economic support of families. Our approach was also unlike that of adult development researchers who have studied fatherhood's influence on men's psychological development. Recruitment and retention have been particularly challenging for the studies reported in this Special Issue because recruitment efforts for the National Early Head Start Research and Evaluation Project targeted mothers who either were pregnant or had a young infant. Not all fathers were present in the household with mother and child. Despite program efforts to involve fathers, some mothers were unwilling to invite the father's involvement in the Early Head Start program. This tension between mothers and fathers in some families challenged researchers to contact and track mobile fathers over their infants' lives, and it was therefore difficult to obtain high response rates. Although we were able to track enough fathers over repeated measurement time points to analyze changes over time in their involvement, the efforts to locate and contact fathers took considerable resources. Such difficulties are commonplace in studies of low-income families, so much so that the Three City Study (2006) discontinued its father study component because of poor response rates (Coley & Schindler, 2003).

Historically, much of what we know about fathers has been from mothers' reports. Consequently, there is need to focus specifically and systematically on father issues with more direct reports from fathers (Tanfer & Mott, 1998). The studies reported in this Special Issue relied primarily on data collected directly from fathers. That said, many of our interview questions were originally developed for mothers; thus, the findings may still lack the precision needed to reveal the full story of fathers. Ryan et al. (this issue) report behaviors of both fathers and mothers when interacting with their children, as directly observed by researchers. This data collection method is important, as it gives researchers directly observed data on parental supportiveness, intrusiveness, detachment, and both negative and positive regard, but even these behaviors were selected based on what is known of mothers' contributions to development and were rated based on past research on the range of mother's behaviors.

The measurement tools needed to penetrate the meaning of paternal beliefs and actions have lagged behind those designed for mothers because scholars are just beginning to define distinct dimensions of the fathering role (Cherlin & Griffith, 1998). The modest, inconsistent relations observed between paternal behavior and child functioning may, to some extent, be an artifact of the lingering use of procedures more appropriate for mothers. Perhaps the rich descriptions offered by the fathers in the Summers et al. (this issue) article may help to address gaps in the measurement of fathering behavior. Fathers' own narrative descriptions of their involvement and their views of the fathering role (Summers et al., this issue) provide elaboration of their self-reports of their interactions with their infants (Shannon et al., this issue) and direct observations of those interactions (Ryan et al., this issue). These rich descriptions also suggest new directions for studying father involvement.

The roles fathers described in more open-ended, qualitative interviews (Summers et al., this issue) suggest domains for future measurement of how fathers provide unique sources of stability and physical interaction not typically studied in mothers, in addition to their own styles of teaching and emotional support that are traditionally observed in mothers. The more flexible approach to descriptions of father involvement such as took place in the qualitative component of the father's studies might eventually result in a tighter definition of fathering that would then reveal tighter links to children's outcomes. Some of this flexibility is evidenced in more extensive qualitative interviews and from unstructured observations of father – child interactions with the fathers in these studies that have not yet been fully analyzed.

Perhaps the most daunting challenge to our research with fathers has been the lack of a tight theoretical perspective to generate hypotheses and guide our methodological approaches to studying key aspects of fathers and fathering. Conceptual frameworks that are relevant to the lives of real fathers in their current circumstances are badly needed as are theories that can ground methods that are engaging to fathers in a wide variety of contexts. We encourage those studying fathers of infants and young children, whether their participants are in circumstances of poverty or privilege, to develop methods and approaches that involve and engage fathers from the beginning and to contribute to building theories about fathers and their roles across families that take into account their diverse cultures and circumstances.

CONCLUSIONS

Consistent with findings from the Summers et al. (this issue) study, Shannon et al. (this issue) cite numerous studies attesting to fathers' desire to be there for their children at the time of birth and during the early years of life. Some fathers, however, are more likely than others to remain present in their children's lives. Shannon and colleagues found that the fathers who continued "being there" were more likely to be older and more educated, with higher levels of income and a better relationship with the children's mothers — probably in more stable situations. The literature shows that the tendency to be involved wanes with time, but studies in this Special Issue show that a significant percentage of low-income fathers remain productively engaged with their children at least through age 3. The studies in this Special Issue also demonstrate that the quality of parenting observed in fathers is connected to the quality of the circumstances surrounding family life (Fitzgerald et al., this issue). High-risk conditions that produce harsh parenting in fathers also produce depression in fathers and higher levels of family conflict.

The continuing macrolevel changes in American culture, together with the volatility that often pervades life among the poor, make it likely that fatherhood for low-income men will continue to be characterized by a diffusion of responsibilities as members of the family. Nonetheless, principles of dynamic systems theory foretell occasional nexus nodes in which fathering behavior and child functioning will come together. Many low-income fathers have a quite clear sense of their role within the family and a considerable impact on their children's adaptive functioning. Likewise, some programs are finding good success in connecting with fathers and meeting their parenting needs. To bring these patterns into clearer resolution against a background of inconsistent associations may require that researchers spend more time investigating nonlinear relations and interaction effects. It may also be of benefit to consider the use of more person-centered approaches to analysis and to examine the impact of change over time. A good example of the latter was intimated in the findings by Shannon et al. (this issue); namely, that children of fathers whose parenting improved from 6 to 14 months showed better self-regulation. Finally, it is important to reiterate what several of the authors in this Special Issue stipulated as a potential limitation for their studies: findings pertaining to father behavior and father effects may be a bit optimistic in that almost all the studies involved use of selective samples — presumably men with greater interest in their children and their own roles as fathers.

The articles in this Special Issue cannot fully answer the questions that drove the Early Head Start team of researchers to include a father component in the national study, and they cannot fully adjudicate the debate about the role of fathers in low-income families, whether as essential contributors to infant development or only as sources of financial support. However, these studies, along with others focused on low-income fathers, should help point the way to more incisive studies of this diverse group of American families who often live in unstable and adverse circumstances.

AFFILIATIONS AND ADDRESSES

Robert H. Bradley, Center for Applied Studies in Education, University of Arkansas at Little Rock, 2801 S. University Avenue, Little Rock, AR 72204–1099. E-mail: rhbradley@ualr.edu. Jeffrey K. Shears is at Colorado State University. Lori A. Roggman is at Utah State University. Catherine S. Tamis-LeMonda is at New York University.

REFERENCES

Bader, A. P. (1995). Engrossment revisited: Fathers are still falling in love with their newborn babies. In J. L. Shapiro, M. J. Diamond, & N. M. Greenberg (Eds.), *Becoming a father* (pp. 224–233). New York: Springer.

Bloom, B. S. (1964). *Stability and change in human characteristics.* New York: Wiley.

Cherlin, A. J., & Griffith, J. (1998). Report of the working group on the methodology of studying fathers. In *Nurturing fatherhood: Improving data and research on male fertility, family formation and fatherhood.* Washington, DC: U.S. Government Printing Office.

Coley, R. L., & Schindler, H. (2003, November). *Measuring father involvement in the Three City Study.* Invited address, Measurement Issues in Family Demography Conference, Bethesda, MD.

Darling, N., & Steinberg, L. (1993). Parenting style as context: An integrative model. *Psychological Bulletin, 113,* 487–496.

England, P., & Folbre, N. (2002). Involving dads: Parental bargaining and family well-being. In C. S. Tamis-LeMonda & N. Cabrera (Eds.), *Handbook of father inolvement* (pp. 387–408). Mahwah, NJ: Lawrence Erlbaum Associates, Inc.

Graham, J. W. & Beller, A. H. (2002). Nonresident fathers and their children: Child support and visitation from an economic perspective. In C. S. Tamis-LeMonda & N. Cabrera (Eds.), *Handbook of father Involvement* (pp. 432–454). Mahwah, NJ: Lawrence Erlbaum Associates, Inc.

Hofferth, S. L., Stueve, J. L., Pleck, J., Bianchi, S., & Sayer, L. (2002). The demography of fathers: What fathers do. In C. S. Tamis-LeMonda & N. Cabrera (Eds.), *Handbook of father involvement, multidisciplinary perspectives* (pp. 63–92). Mahwah, NJ: Lawrence Erlbaum Associates, Inc.

Lamb, M. E. (1997). Fathers and child development: An introductory overview and guide. In M. E. Lamb (Ed.), *The role of the father in child development* (pp. 1–18). New York: Wiley.

Lamb, M. E. (2000). The history of research on father involvement: An overview. *Marriage & Family Review, 29,* 23–42.

Lamb, M. E. (2002). Nonresidential fathers and their children. In C. S. Tamis-LeMonda & N. Cabrera (Eds.), *Handbook of father involvement* (pp. 169–184). Mahwah, NJ: Lawrence Erlbaum Associates, Inc.

Mincy, R. B., & Pouncy, H. W. (2002). The responsible fatherhood field: Evolution and goals. In C. S. Tamis-LeMonda & N. Cabrera (Eds.), *Handbook of father involvement, multidisciplinary perspectives* (pp. 555–597). Mahwah, NJ: Lawrence Erlbaum Associates, Inc.

Palkovitz, R. (2002). Involved fathering and child development: Advancing our understanding of good fathering. In C. S. Tamis-LeMonda & N. Cabrera (Eds.), *Handbook of father involvement* (pp. 119–140). Mahwah, NJ: Lawrence Erlbaum Associates, Inc.

Parke, R. D. (2002). Fathers and families. In M. H. Bornstein (Ed.), *Handbook of parenting, Vol. 3: Being and becoming a parent* (2nd ed., pp. 27–73). Mahwah, NJ: Lawrence Erlbaum Associates, Inc.

Rodholm, M., & Larsson, K. (1982). The behavior of human adults at their first contact with a newborn. *Infant Behavior and Development, 5,* 121–130.

Tanfer, K. & Mott, F. (1998). The meaning of fatherhood for men. In *Nurturing fatherhood: Improving data and research on male fertility, family formation and fatherhood* (pp. 249–293). Washington, DC: U.S. Government Printing Office.

Three City Study. (2006). Retrieved February 13, 2006, from http://www.nichd.nih.gov/about/cpr/dbs/res_three.htm

Yogman, M. (1981). Games fathers and mothers play with their infants. *Infant Mental Health Journal, 2,* 241–248.

EDITORIAL SCOPE

Parenting: Science and Practice strives to promote the exchange of empirical findings, theoretical perspectives, and methodological approaches from all disciplines that help to define and advance theory, research, and practice in parenting, caregiving, and childrearing broadly construed. *Parenting: Science and Practice* addresses parents and the role of alternate caregivers who supplement or sometimes substitute for parents. Articles on parenting itself, antecedents of parenting, parenting effects on parents and on children, the multiple contexts of parenting, and parenting interventions and education are welcome. The journal is committed to enriching our understanding of parenting in all its manifestations.

Parenting: Science and Practice is an international and interdisciplinary peer-reviewed journal that seeks to publish rigorous empirical, methodological, applied, review, theoretical, perspective, and policy pieces relevant to parenting; contributions from the humanities and biological sciences as well as the social sciences are invited. The journal will also publish notices of books and other publications or media representations relevant to the study of parenting.

Departments

Parenting: Science and Practice has five main departments: Inquiries about prospective submissions to any department should be addressed to the Editor.

- **Empirical Articles.** The journal is principally committed to the publication of empirical articles. Creative, comprehensive, and clear reports that advance the empirical base and theory in the field of parenting studies are sought, and all modes of empirical research are welcome: experimental, observational, ethnographic, textual, interpretive, and survey.
- **Reviews.** Reviews of the literature may be empirically grounded or theoretical; they should be scholarly, integrative, and timely, synthesizing or evaluating an issue relevant to parenting. Published reviews are normally accompanied by a small number of solicited commentaries from specialists in parenting as well as in allied fields.
- **Statements.** Statements published in *Parenting* provide a forum for the rapid dissemination of new hypotheses, fresh concepts, innovative methods, or emerging trends. Statements should be tightly reasoned and empirically grounded and must be cogent and succinct. Statements should not exceed 3,000 words in length.
- **Tutorials in Parenting.** *Parenting* publishes occasional tutorials that debut new theory in parenting or explore the intersection of parenting with an academic specialty pertinent to parenting studies. These papers define the concept or the field, crystallize its major contributions, detail direct associations with parenting, and augur future directions of application.
- **Media Notices.** Summaries and evaluations of books, periodicals, websites, and other media that concern themselves with parenting studies or practices will appear in the journal. Send relevant material to the Editor.

ADDITIONAL JOURNAL FEATURES

THEMATIC ISSUES

Parenting: Science and Practice welcomes proposals for Thematic Issues. Thematic Issues need to have components that link together closely in some meaningful conceptual or theoretical way, and the proposer of a Thematic Issue becomes the Guest Editor. Thematic Issues may be invited or open competitions, but all submissions must be peer reviewed. Individuals interested in developing a Thematic Issue should send the Editor a brief proposal and justification. Some proposals may be more appropriate for the *Monographs in Parenting* series.

MEDIA NOTICES

Parenting: Science and Practice will publish summaries and evaluations of books, periodicals, websites, and other media that concern themselves with parenting studies and childcare practices. Send relevant material to the Editor.

MONOGRAPHS IN PARENTING

To accompany the journal, *Monographs in Parenting* publishes authored or edited volumes whose central concern is parenting, caregiving, and childrearing broadly construed. Inquiries about potential submissions to the *Monographs in Parenting* series are invited.

AUDIENCE

Parenting: Science and Practice will appeal to scholars and practitioners in psychology, human development, family science, clinical practice, social work, education, pediatrics, psychiatry, sociology, anthropology, demography, and related disciplines. Articles published in *Parenting: Science and Practice* will be meaningful to parents and students as well as researchers and policy makers.

WEBSITE

Parenting: Science and Practice's website provides archival titles and synopses of published papers and supplements the journal with abstracts, tables, audio, video, and other multimedia elements that expand upon articles presented in the journal.

Visit: www.parentingscienceandpractice.com

MANUSCRIPT SUBMISSION

Cover Letter: (1) Include a brief statement that indicates what the study will tell the readership of the journal and indicate the intended department. (2) If submitting an empirical report, warrant that the study was conducted in accordance with the ethical standards of the American Psychological Association (APA). (3) Affirm that all authors are in agreement with the contents of the manuscript.

Submission: (1) Submit by electronic mail to the Editor at the e-mail address given below. (2) The manuscript should include a cover sheet containing the title of the manuscript, the name(s) of the author(s) and affiliation(s), and the street address, telephone, fax, and electronic mail address of the corresponding author. (3) The title of the paper, but not names of the author(s), should appear on the first page of the text. Include a Synopsis following the guidelines set forth in the *Parenting* Style Guide (available at the website or from the Editor). Normally, follow the guidelines on requirements, format, and style provided in the *Publication Manual of the American Psychological Association* (5th ed.); see also *Parenting*'s own Style Guide. The manuscript should be double spaced throughout. Set figures in Book Antiqua. (4) Manuscripts should be written concisely; a manuscript of more than 60 pages may be considered as appropriate for the *Monographs in Parenting* series. (5) Manuscripts may not be submitted simultaneously to *Parenting: Science and Practice* and to other journals. (6) The corresponding author accepts responsibility for informing all coauthors of manuscript submission and editorial decisions.

Review: Manuscripts are reviewed by the Editor, members of the Board of Editors, and invited reviewers with expertise in the area(s) represented by the manuscript. Submissions must be appropriate and of moment to the readership of *Parenting: Science and Practice* and should meet a high level of scientific acceptability. A first level of review determines the appropriateness, import, and scientific merit for the journal; on this basis, the Editor reserves the right to review the manuscript further. The Editor also retains the right to decline manuscripts that do not meet established ethical standards. A system of blind reviewing is used; however, it is the author's responsibility to remove information about the identity of author(s) and affiliation(s) from the body of the manuscript. Such information should appear on the cover sheet. The Editor will have the discretion to integrate solicited reviews into a determinative response.